The Big Book of Animals- Coloring for adults

By

Sassy Angel

Copyright © 2017 Dark Starlight Publications/ Sassy Angel All rights reserved. No part of this publication may be reproduced, distributed, or transmitted in any form or by any means, including photocopying, recording, or other electronic or mechanical methods, without the prior written permission of the publisher, except in the case of brief quotations embodied in critical reviews and certain other noncommercial uses permitted by copyright law. Frist Edition printed in the U.S. A. Please note: This book was written by someone who has a learning disability and couldn't read or write until the age of 16. The author has also suffered a Traumatic brain injury. (TBI) is a form of brain injury caused by sudden damage to the brain. (I got mine from having two strokes) I share this with you not to gain your sympathy but to share and inspire that people with disabilities can do anything they set their mind to. ISBN-13:

978-1977683946 ISBN-10:

1977683940

Introduction

This adult coloring book has over 50 animal patterns and provides hours of stress relief through creative expression. It features small and big creatures from forests, oceans, deserts and grasslands. Designs range in complexity and detail from beginner to expert-level. This book is perfect for anyone with a brain injury, who has Alzheimer's, dementia, PTSD, older adults that want to keep their minds sharp, people with memory issues, or anyone who wants to relive stress. The images are safe for the whole family.

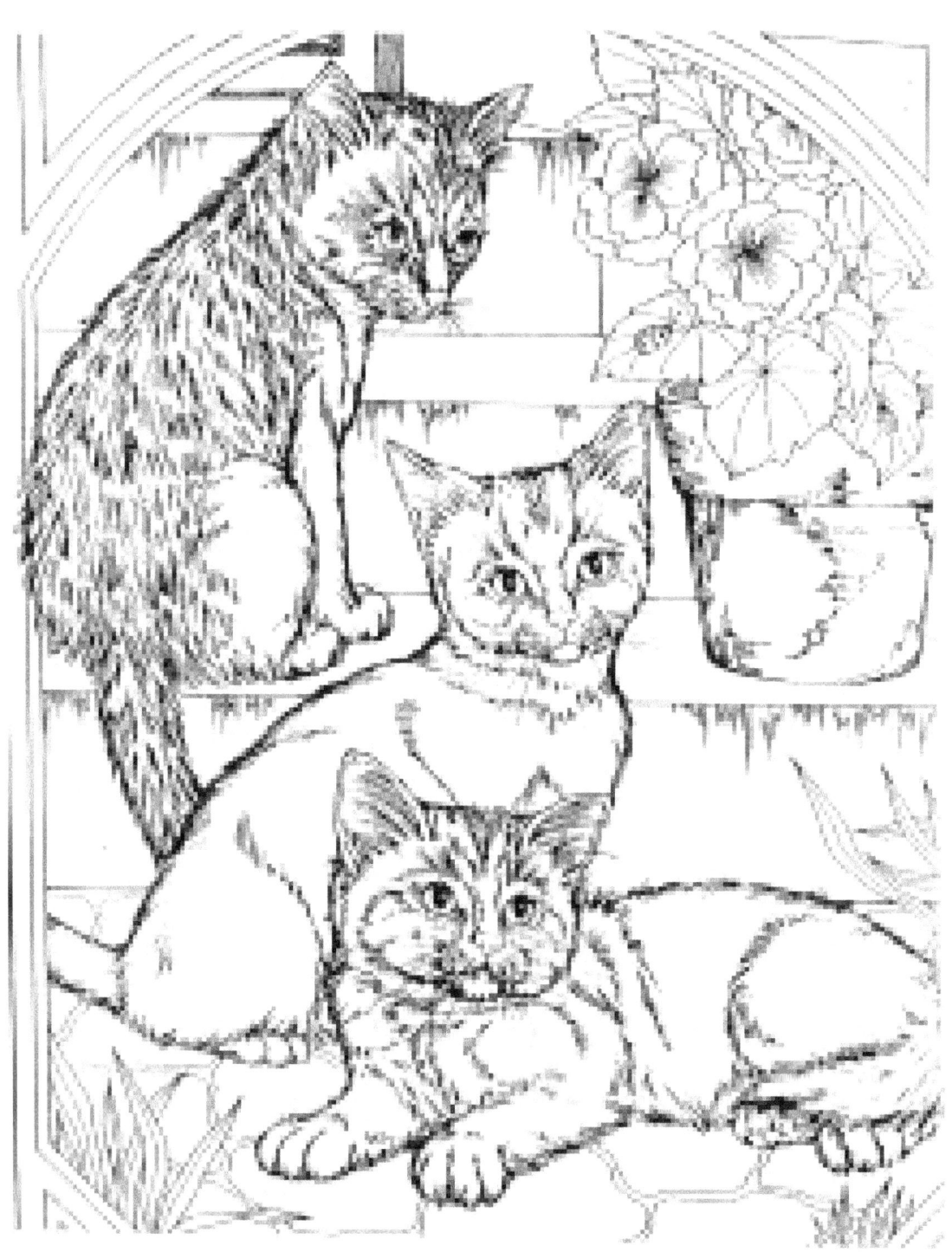

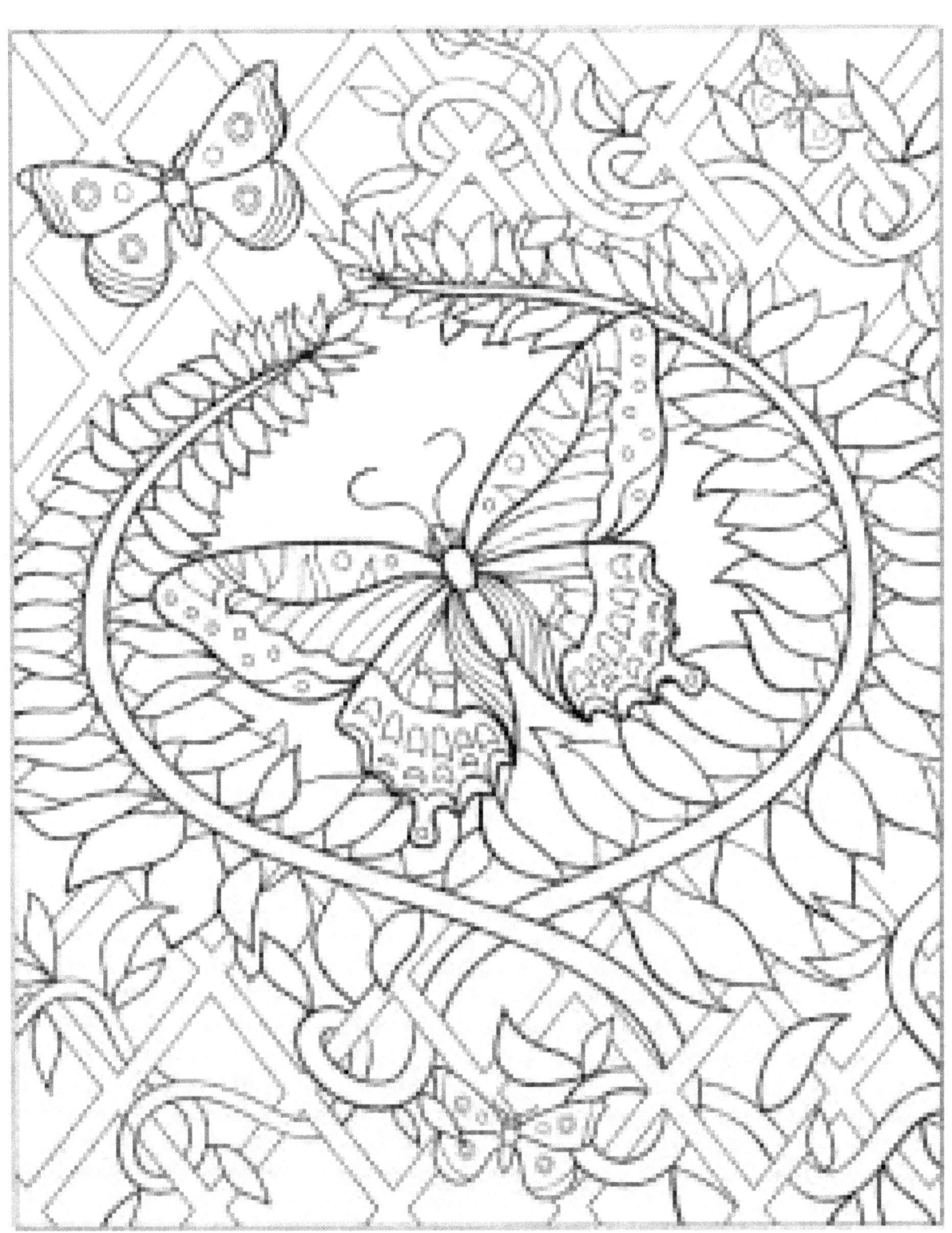

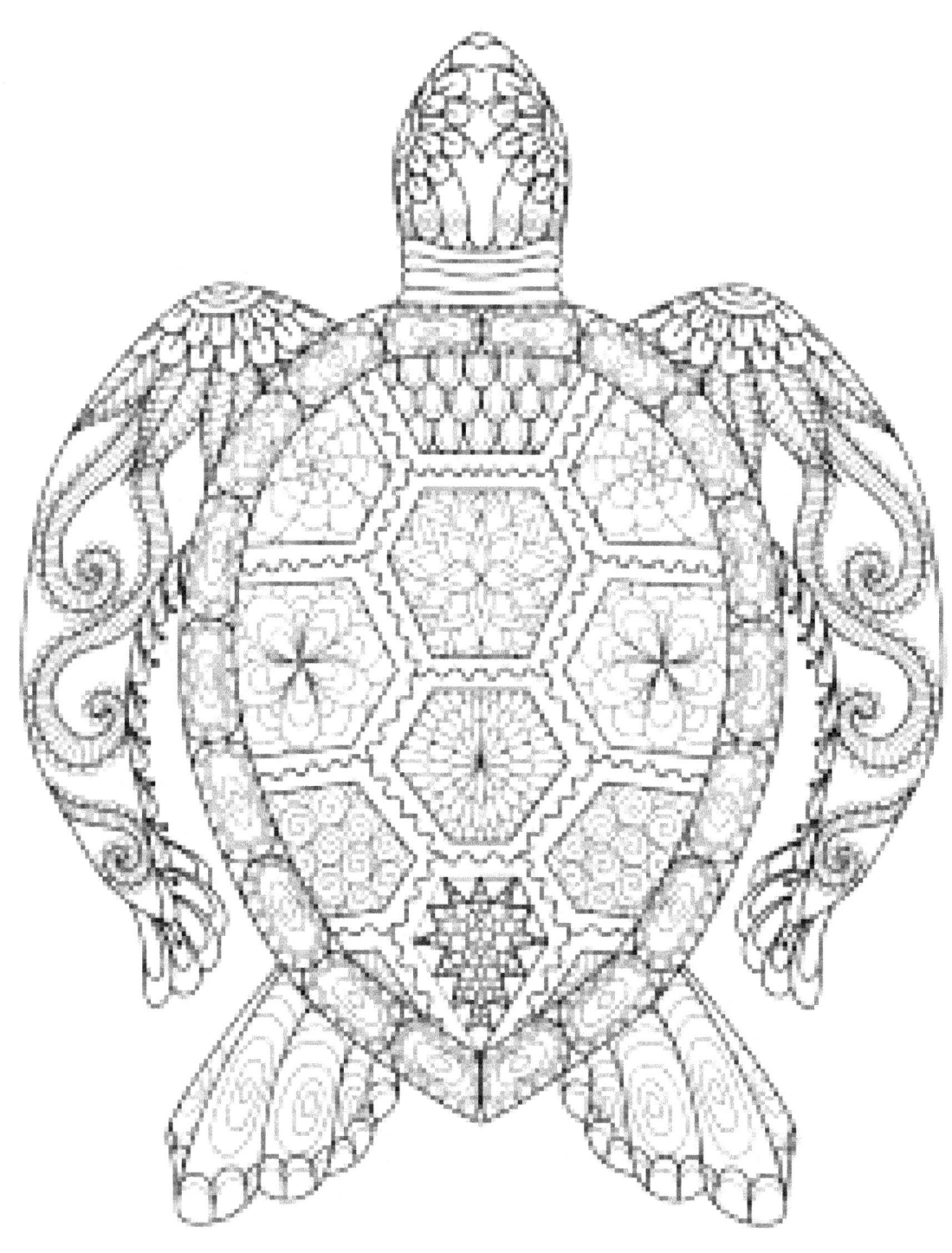

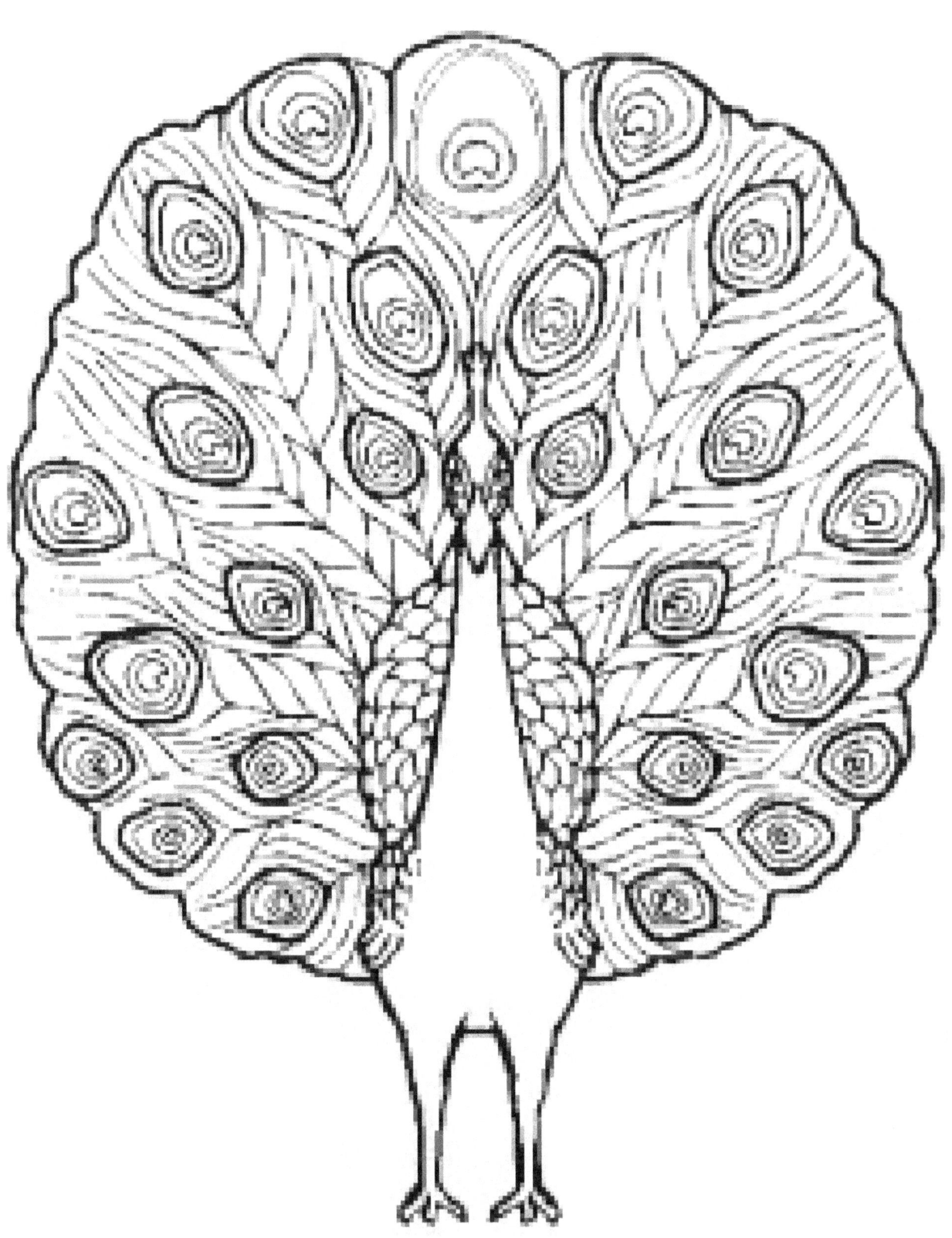

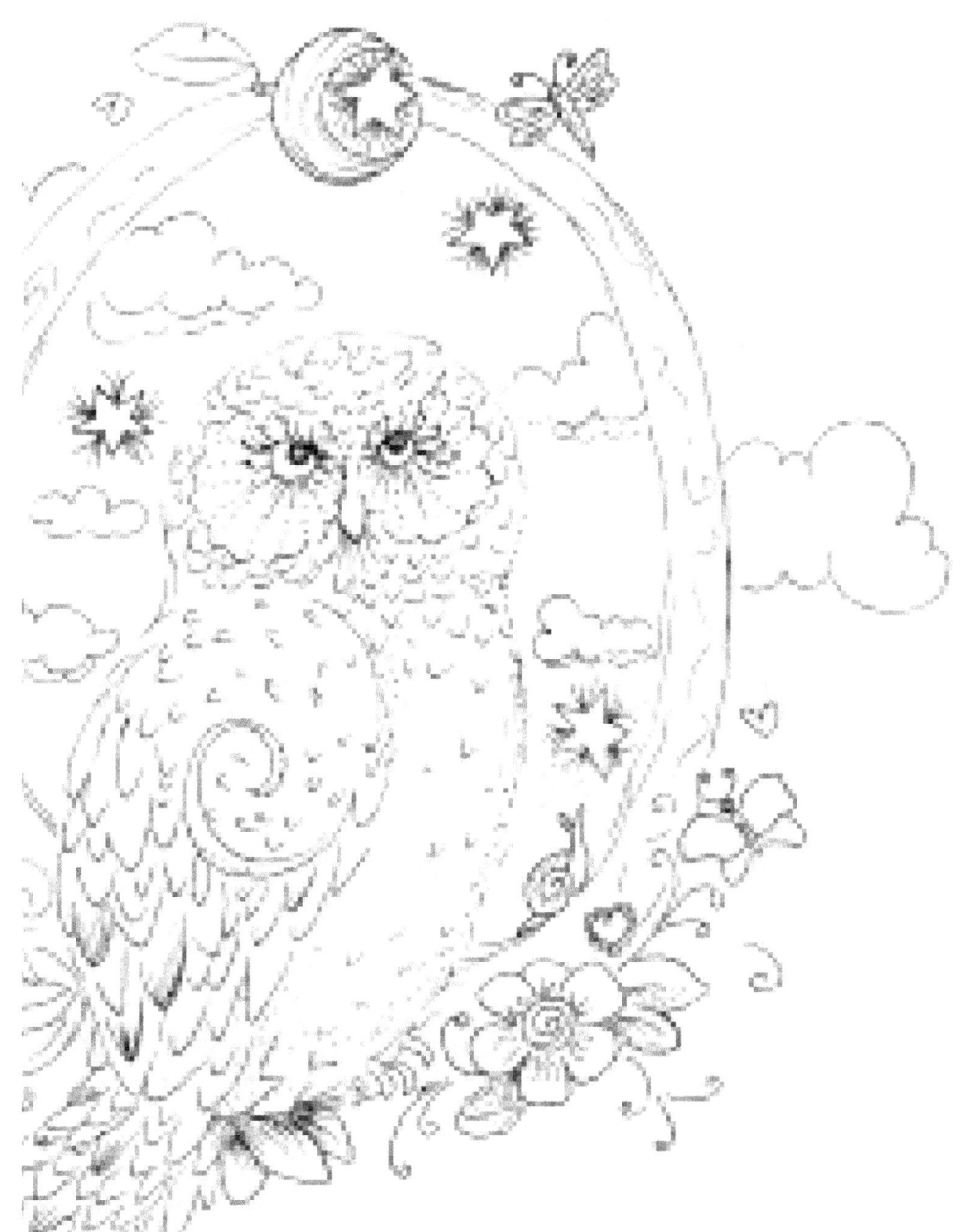

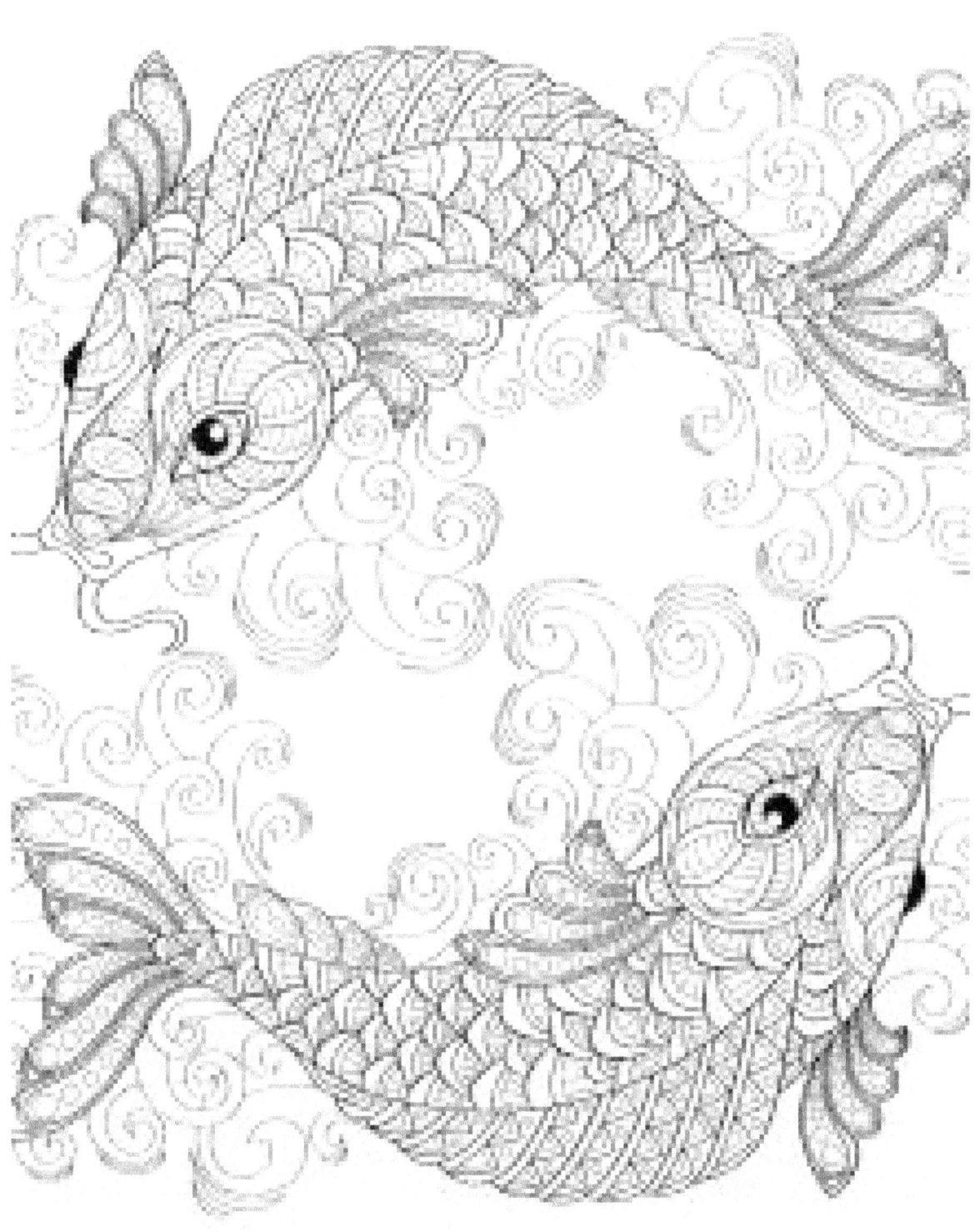

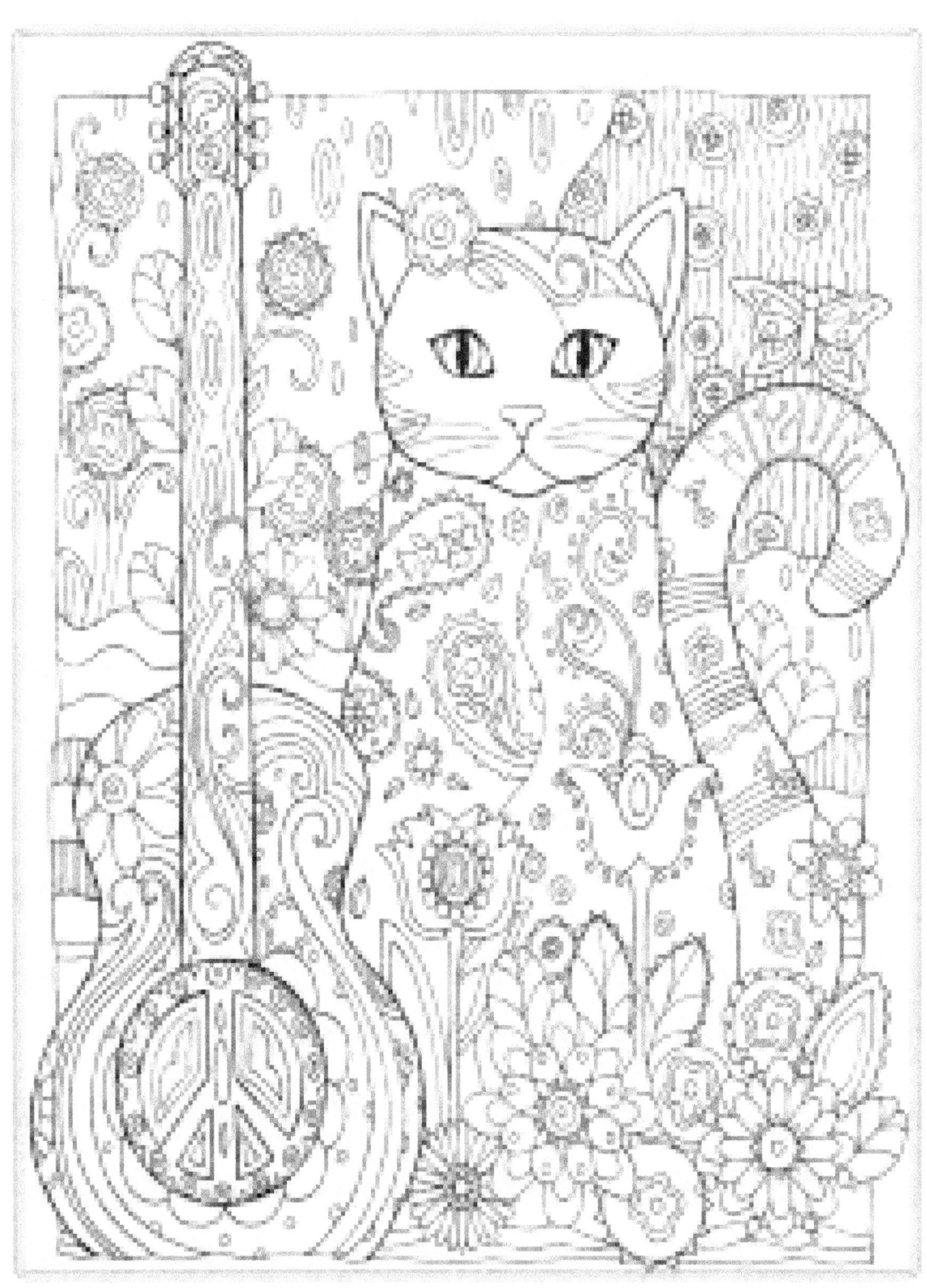

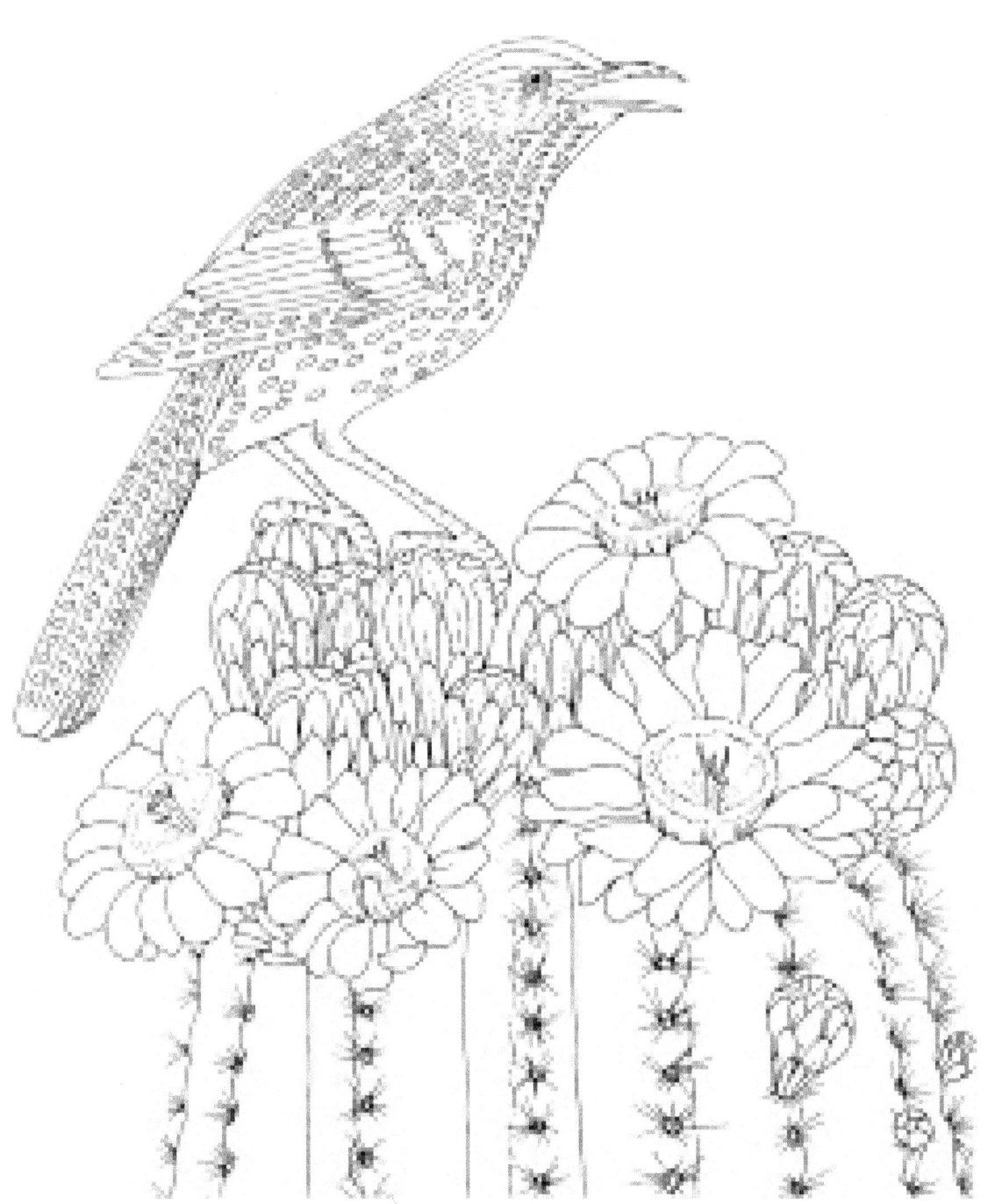

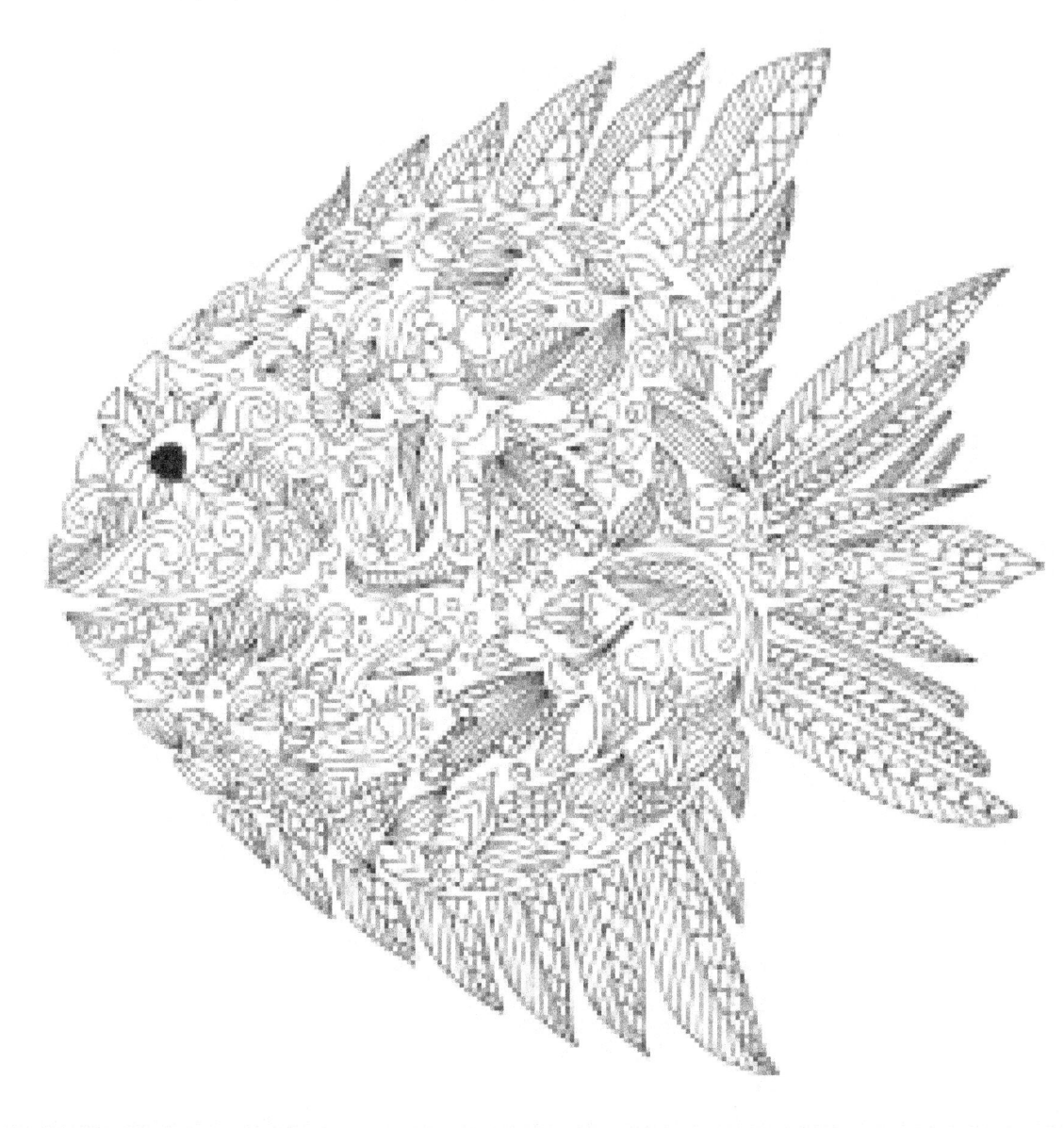

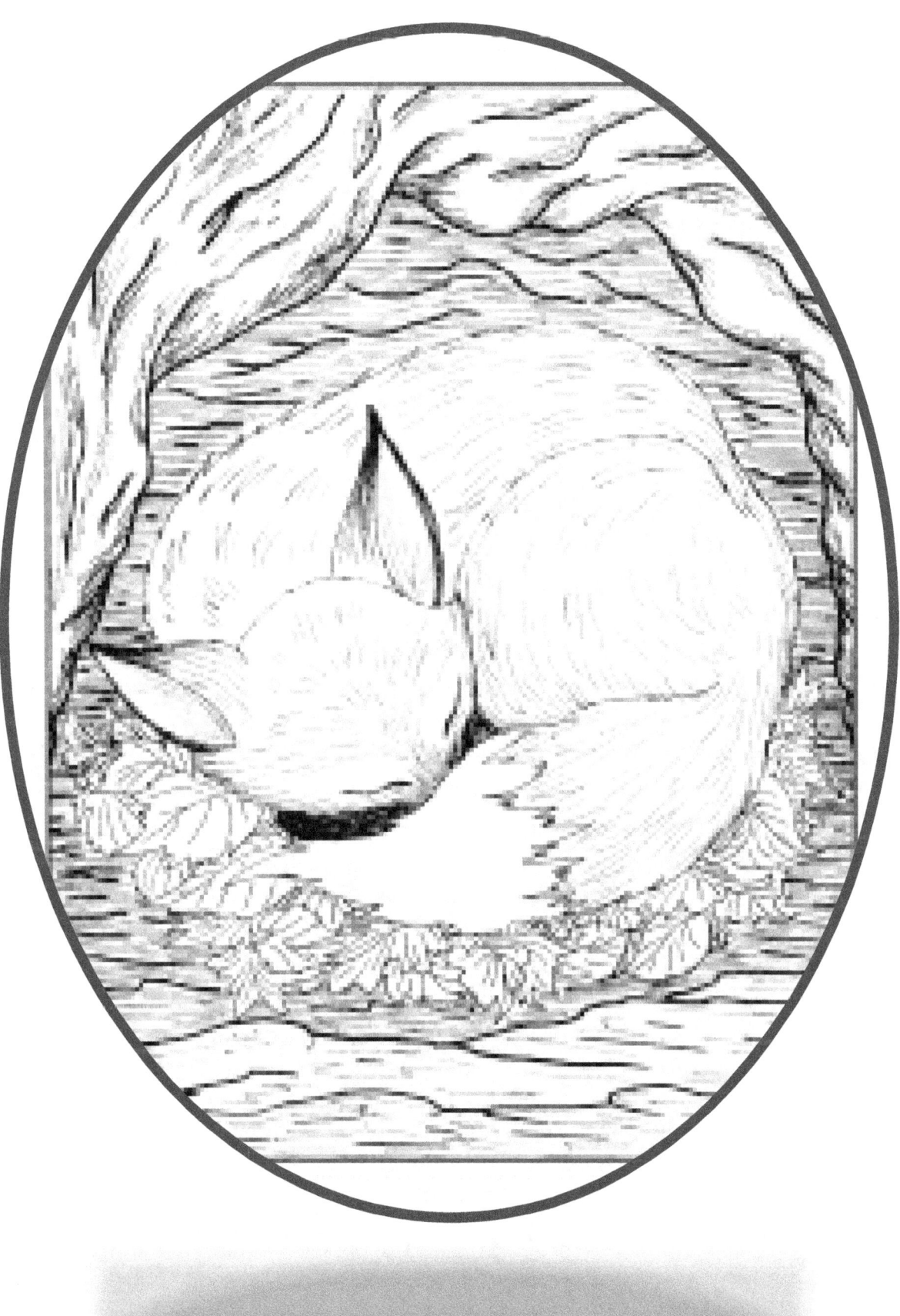

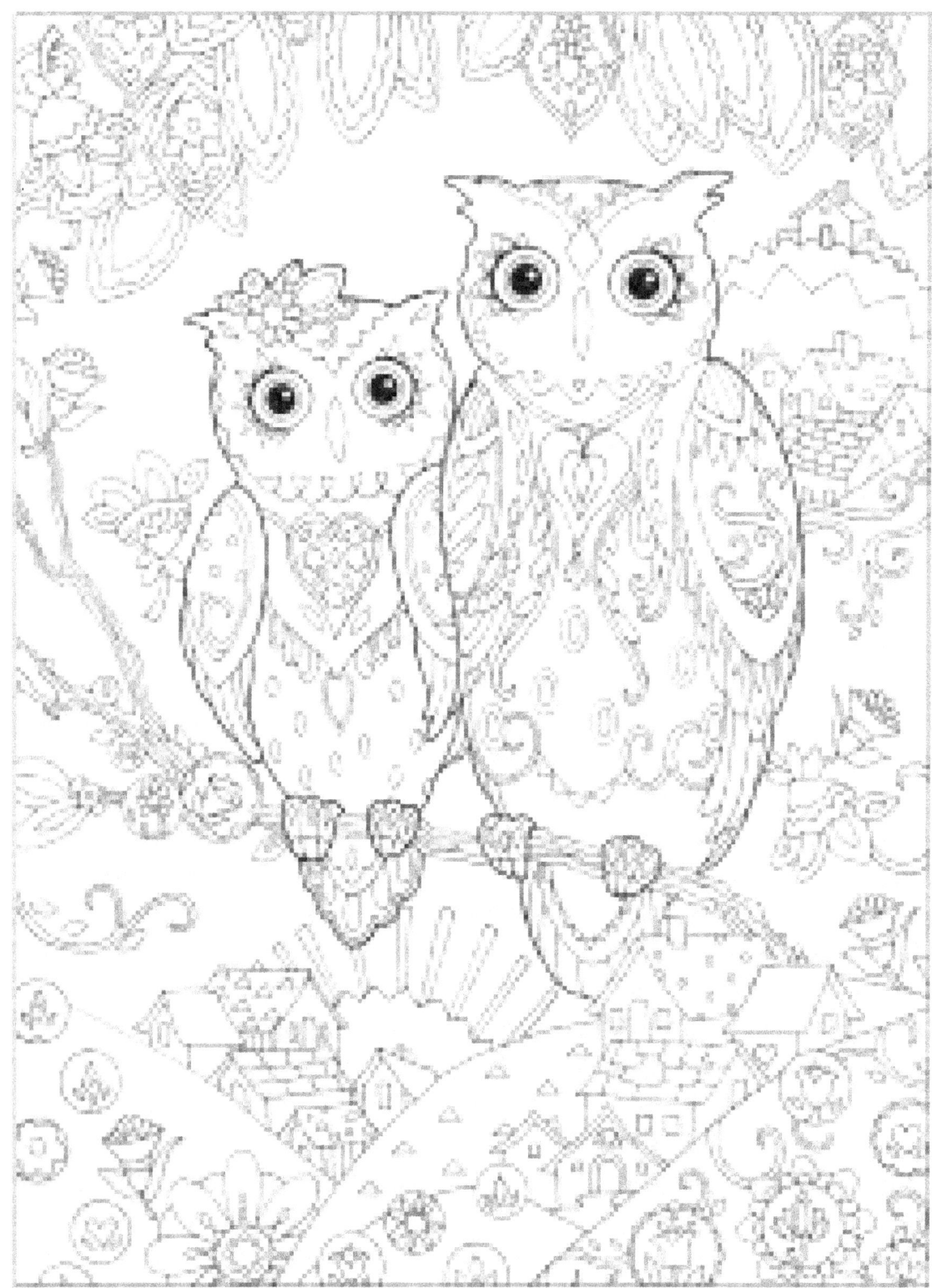

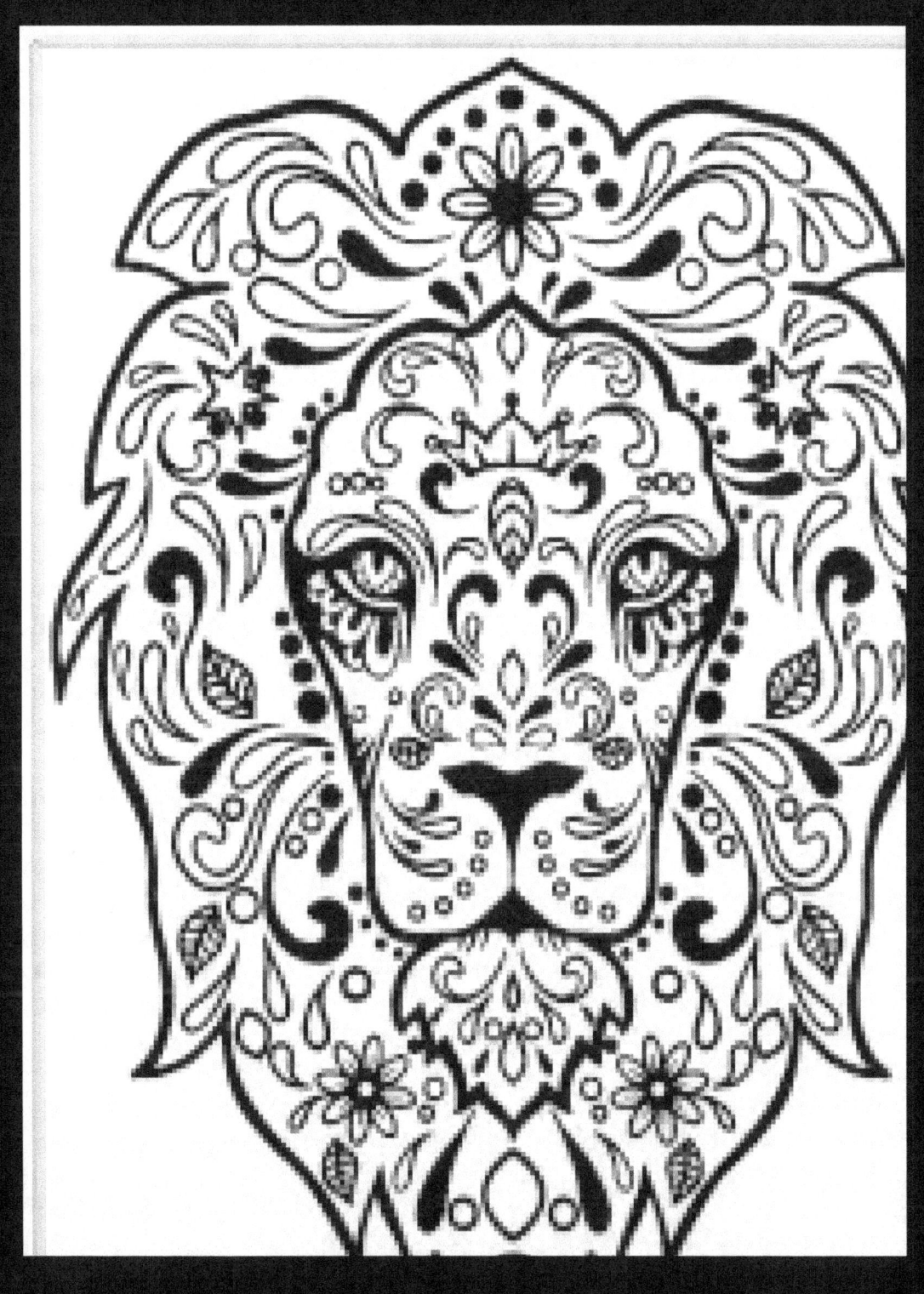

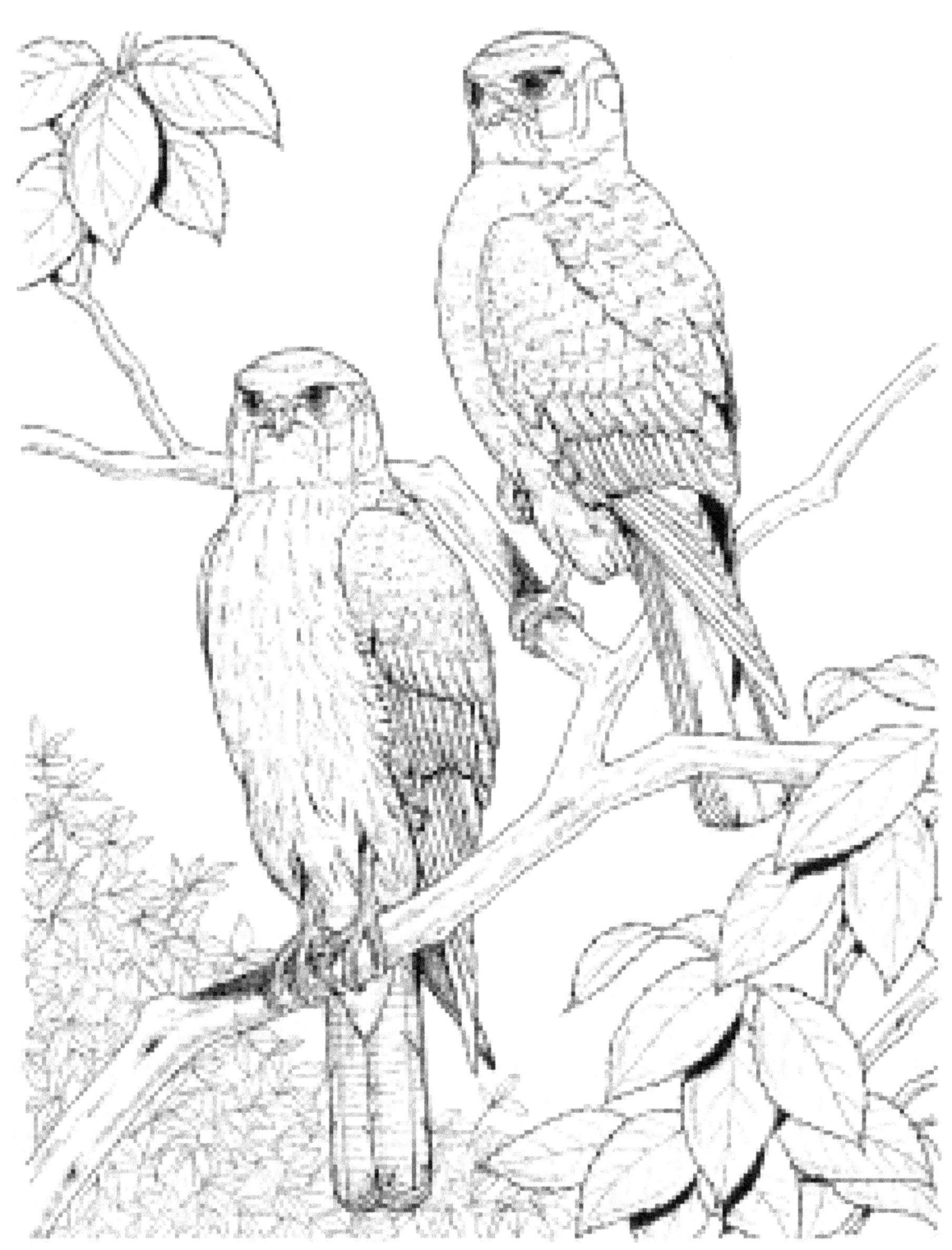

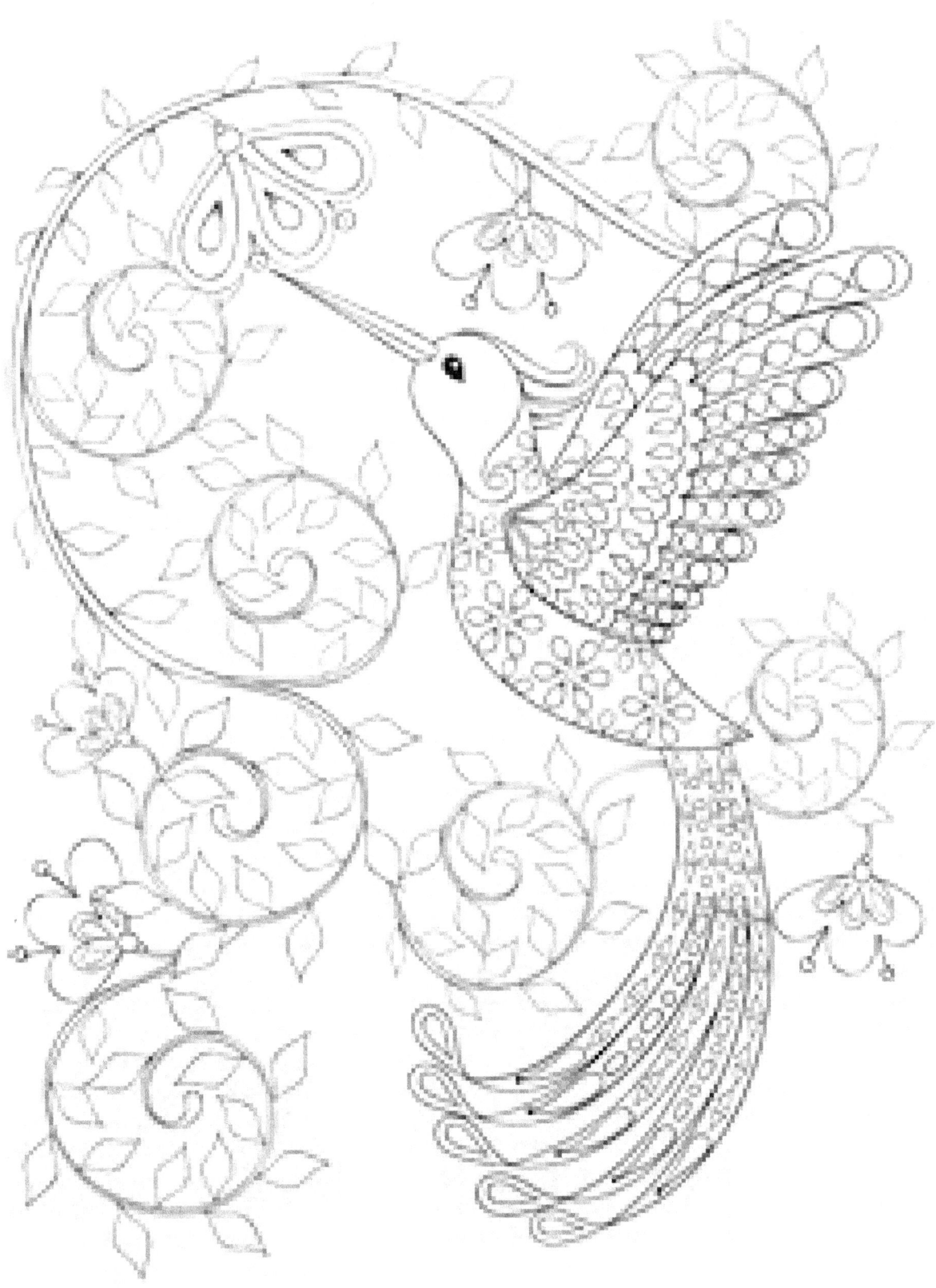

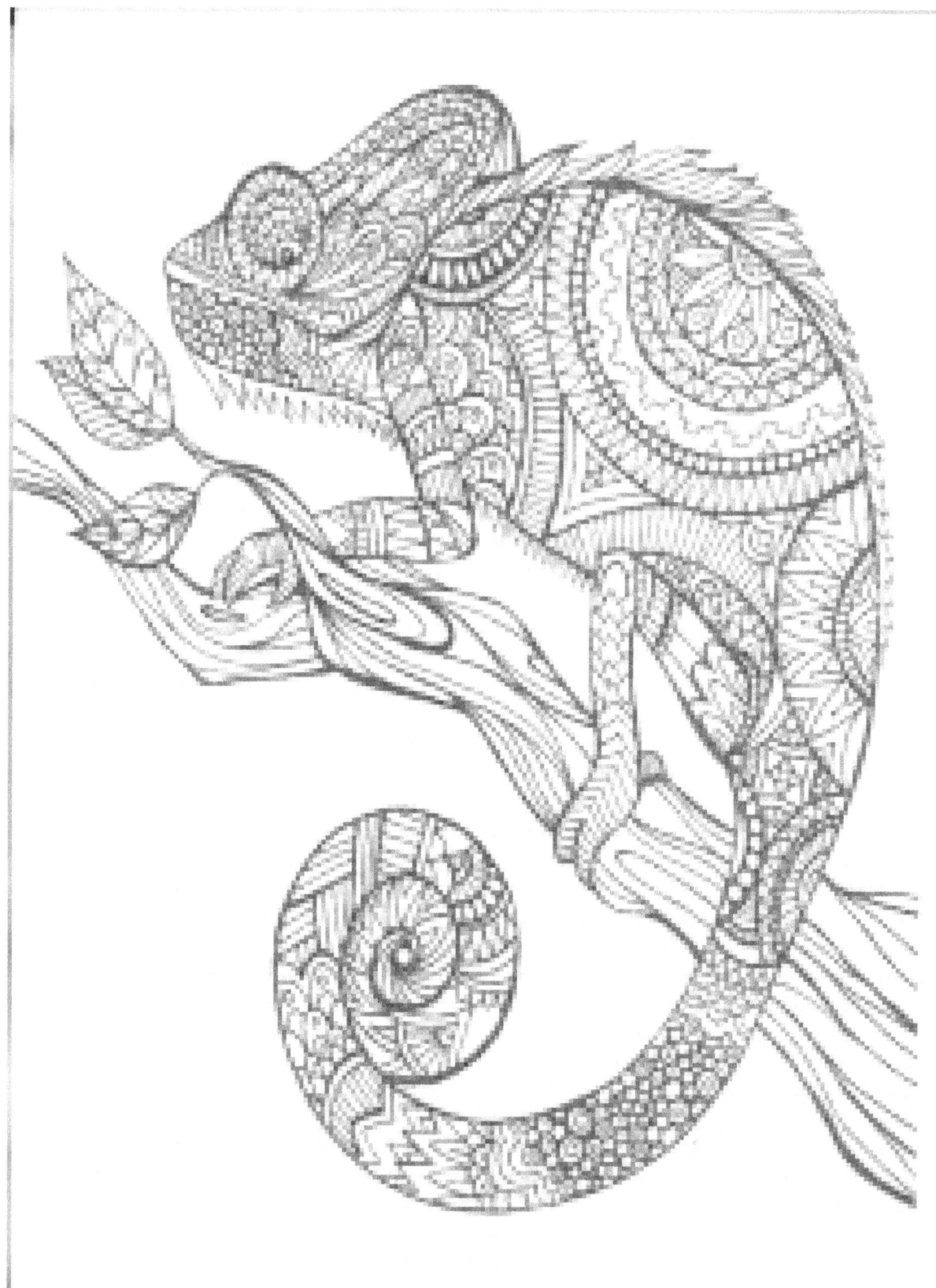

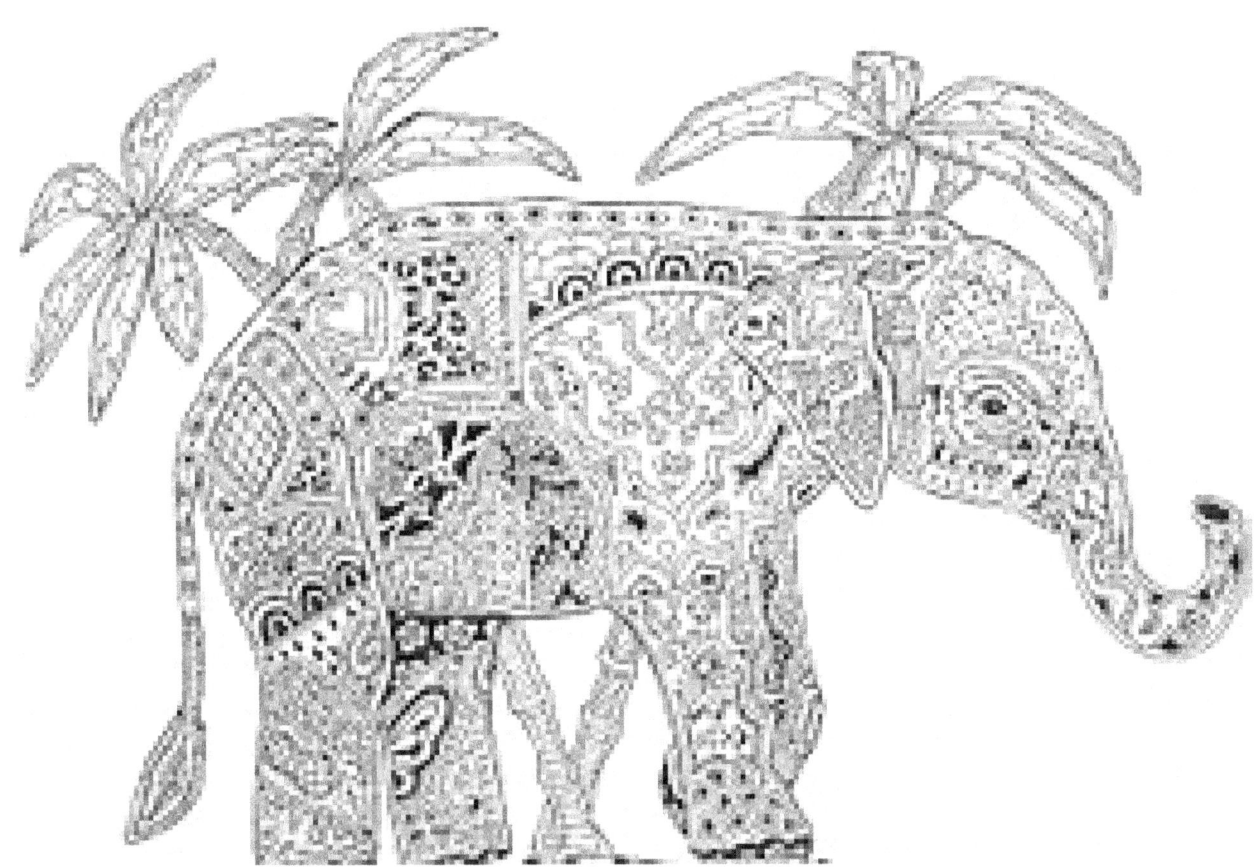

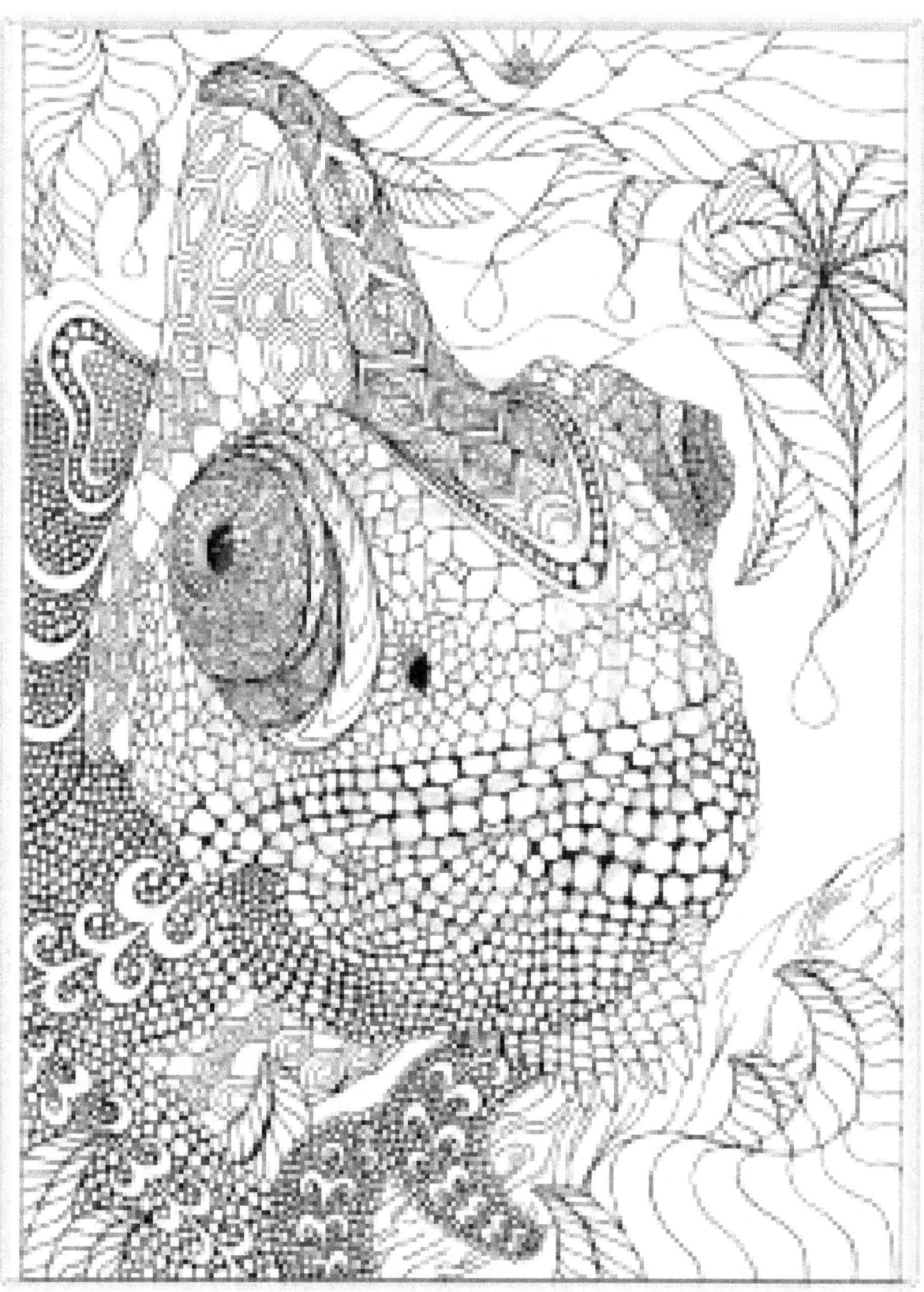

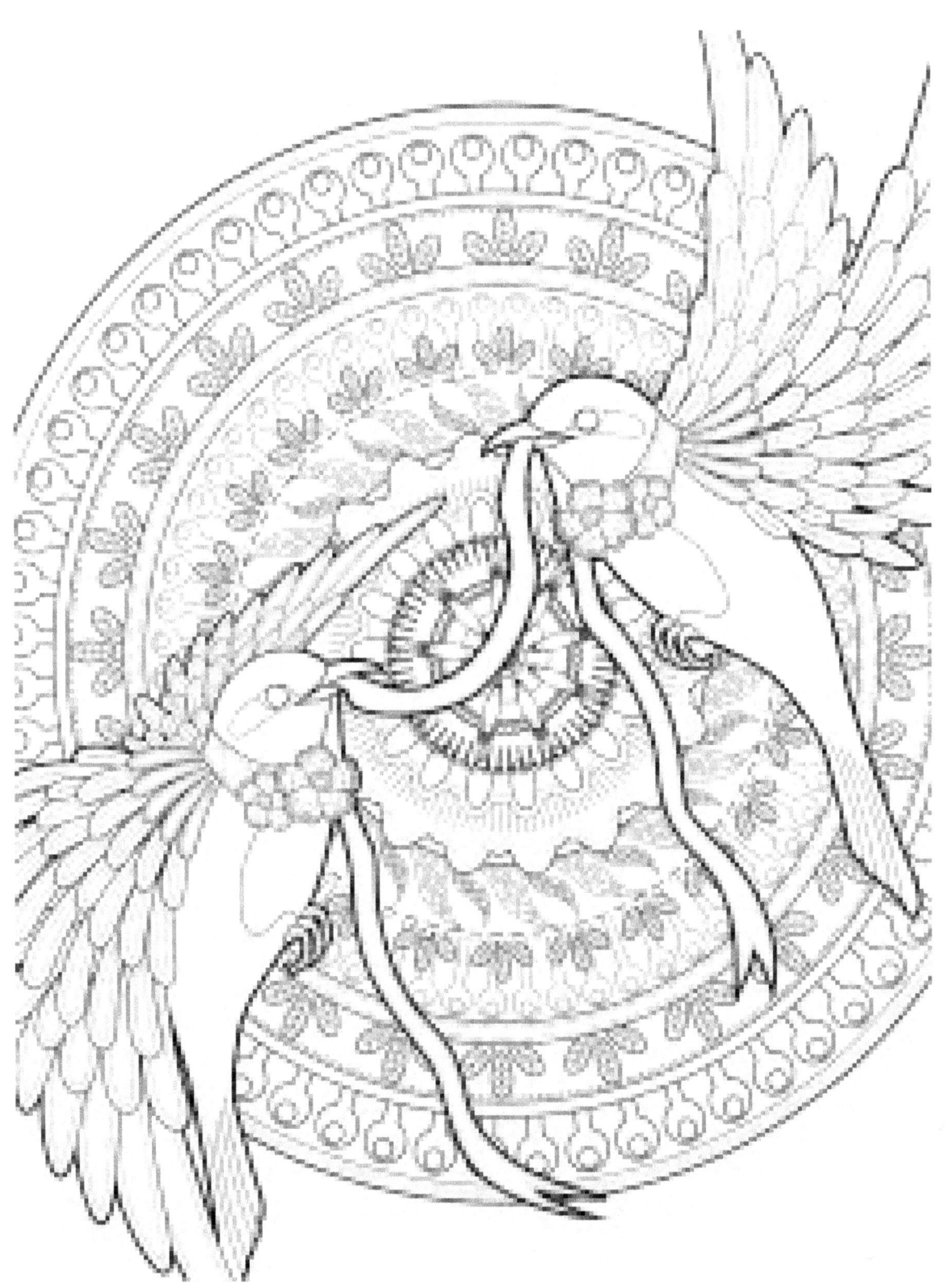

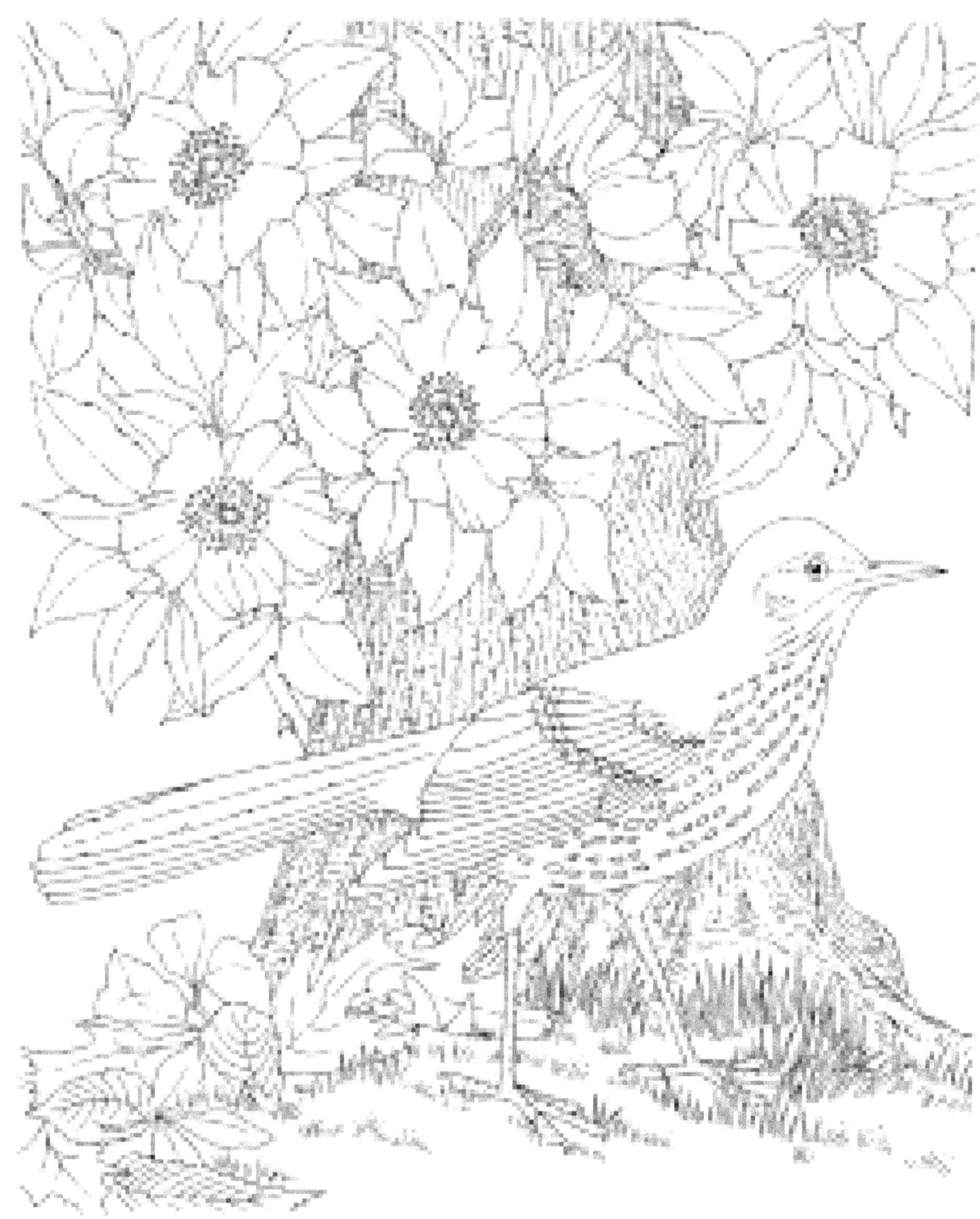

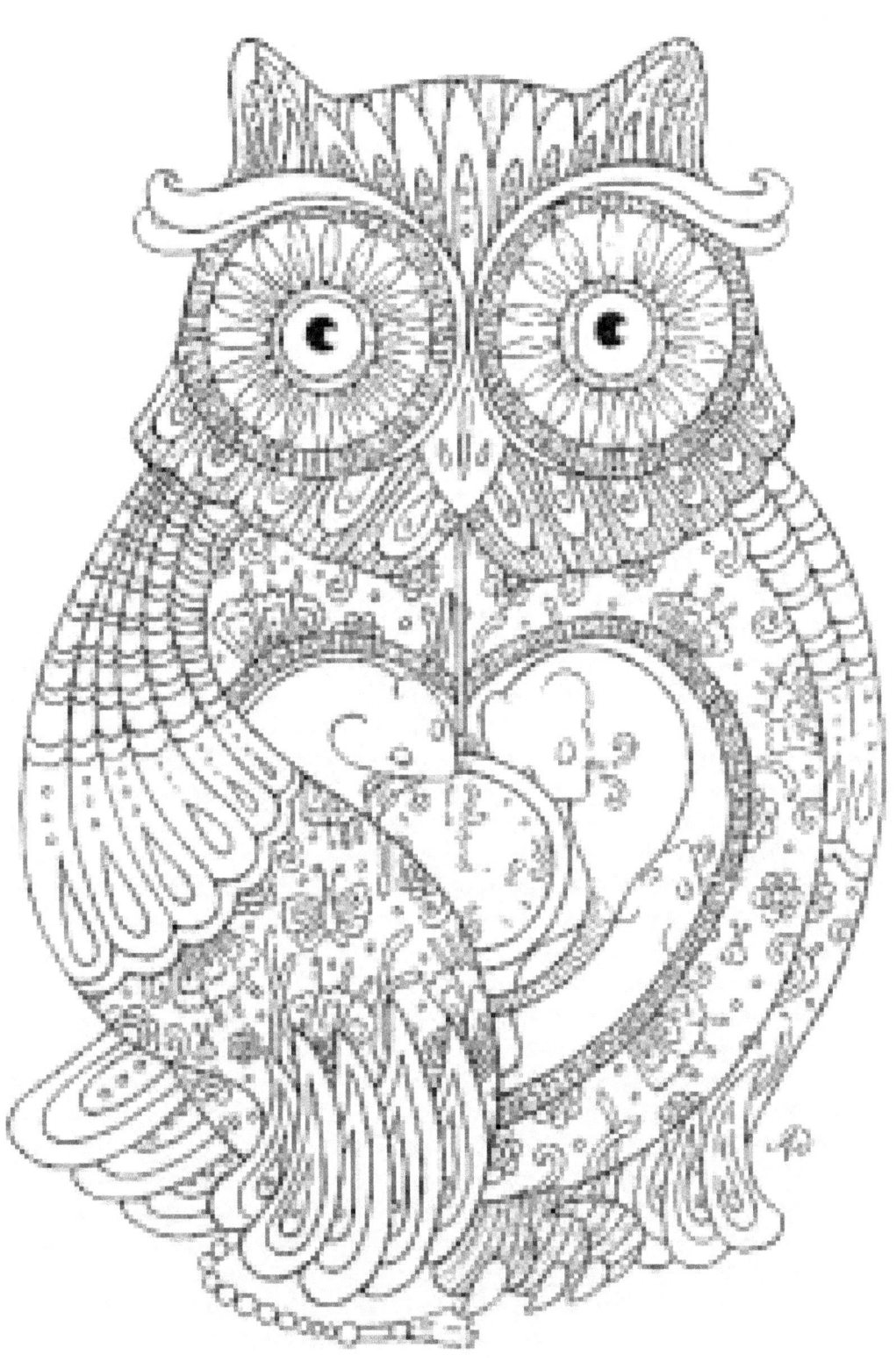

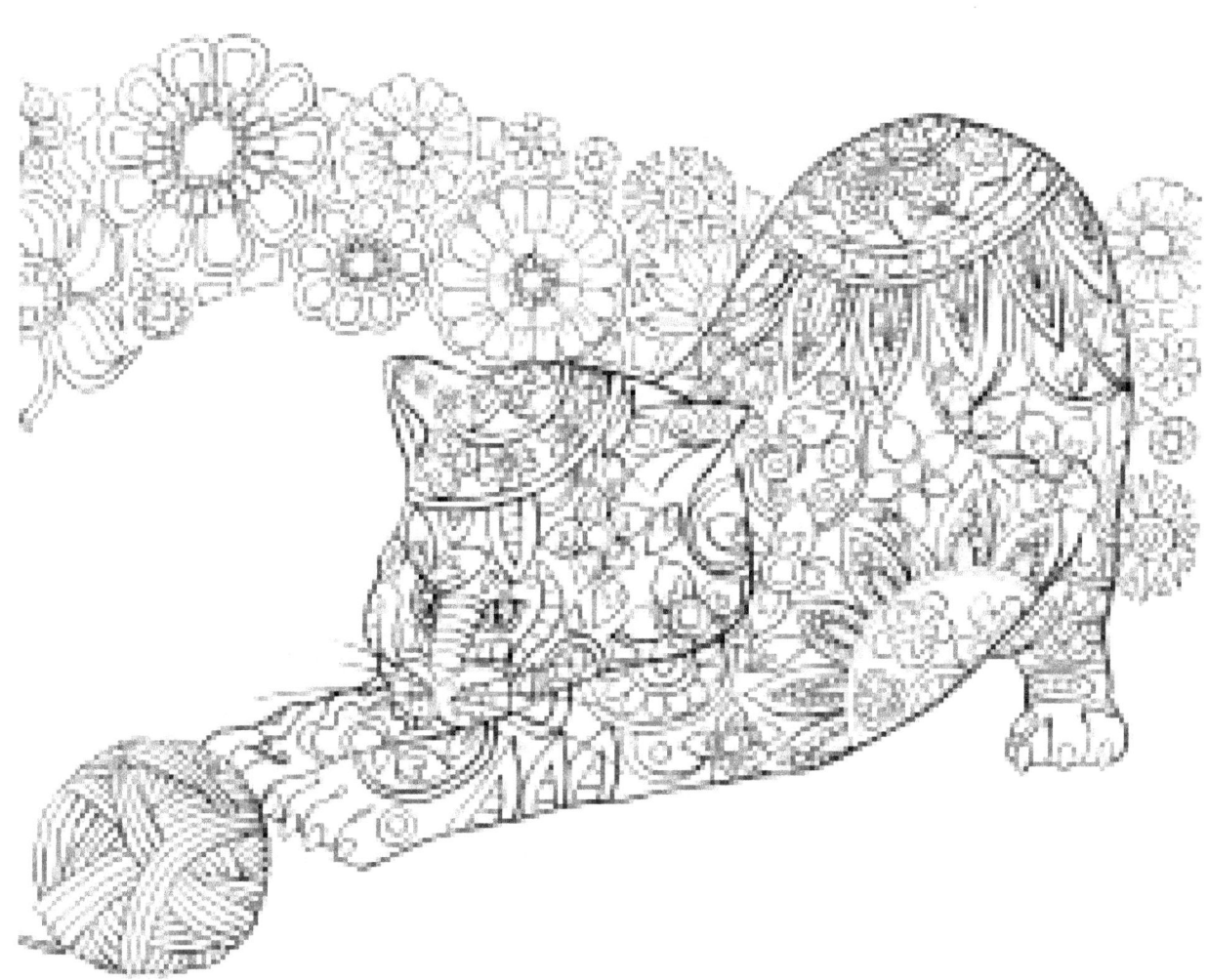

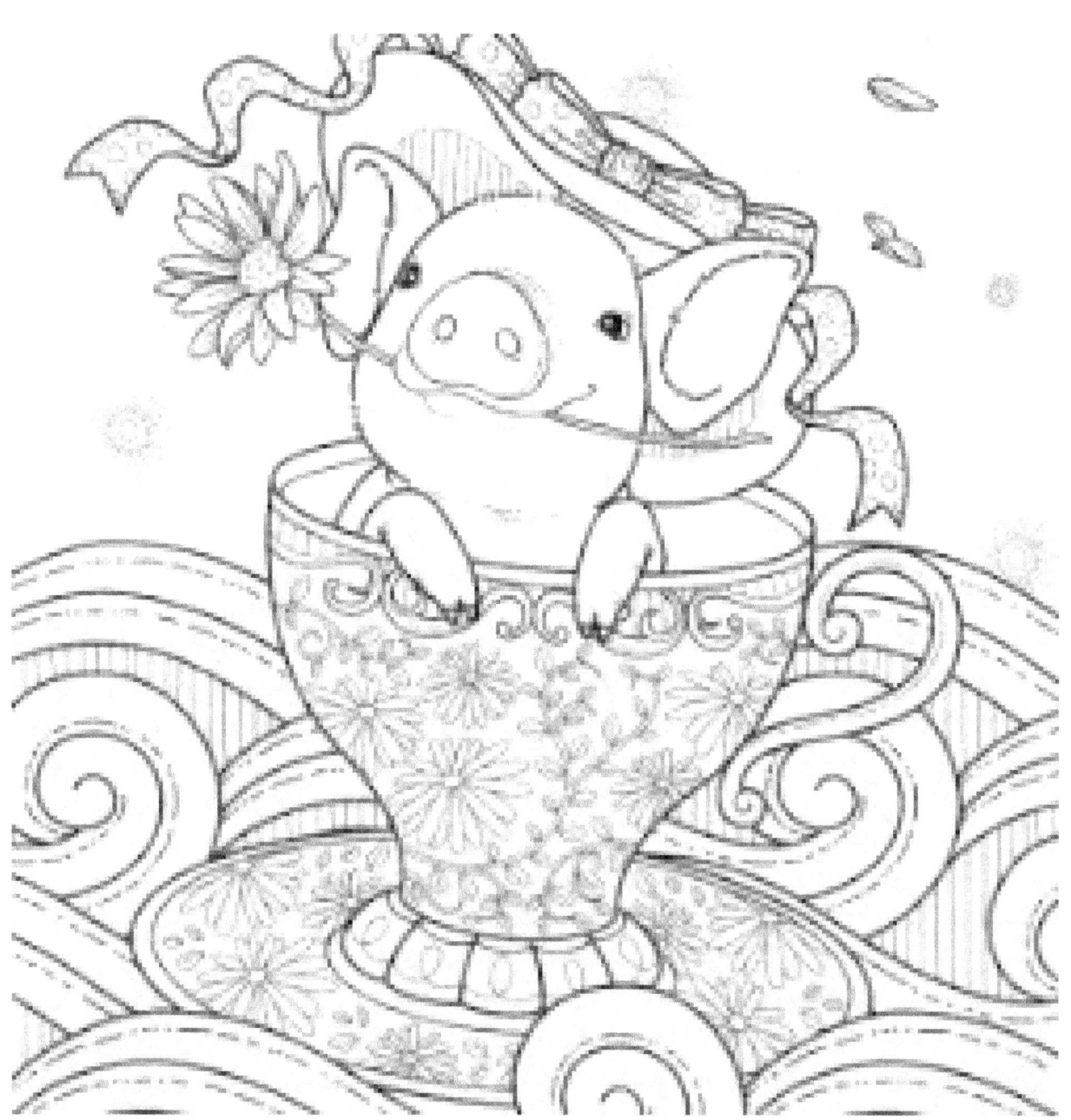

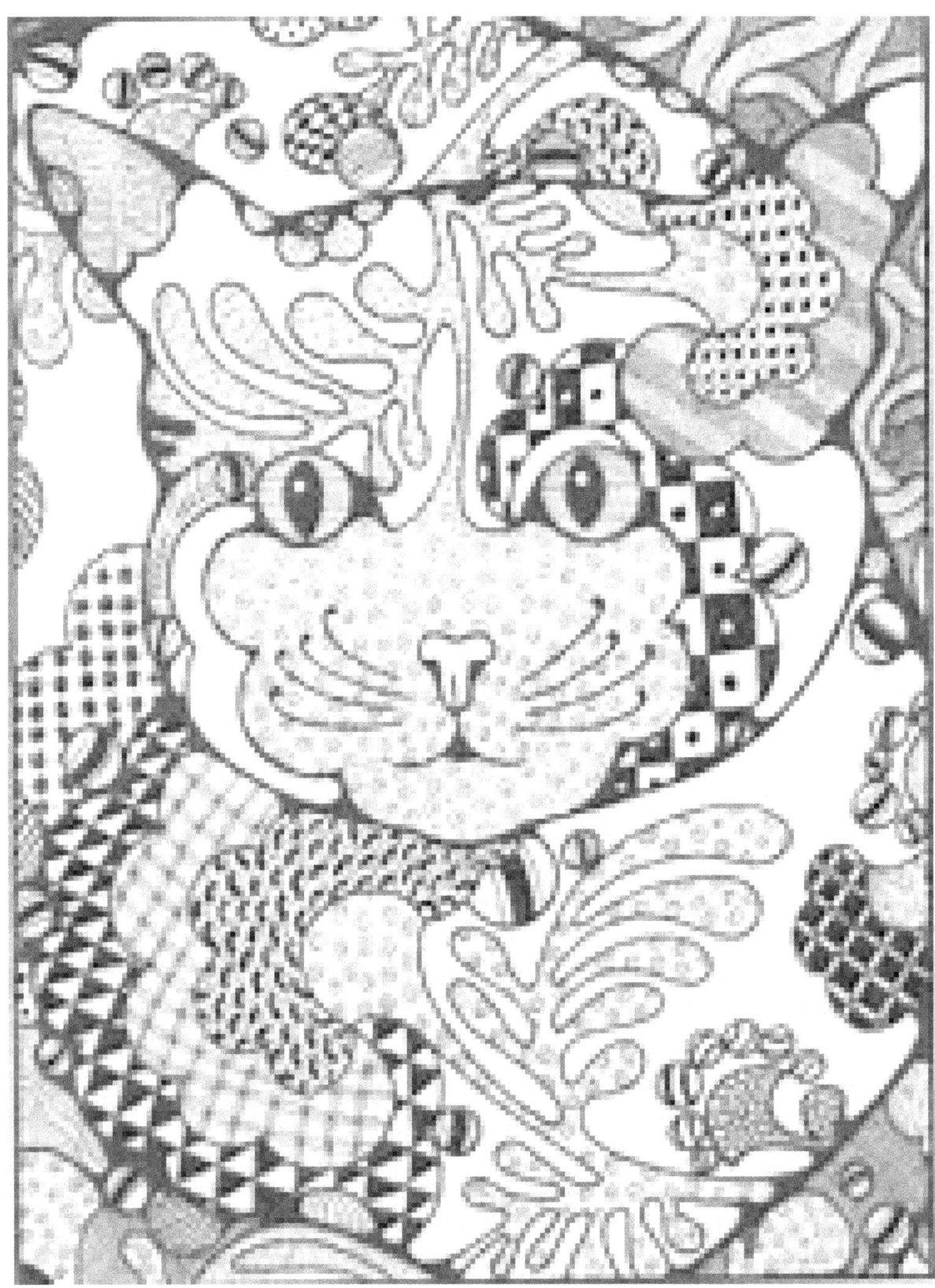

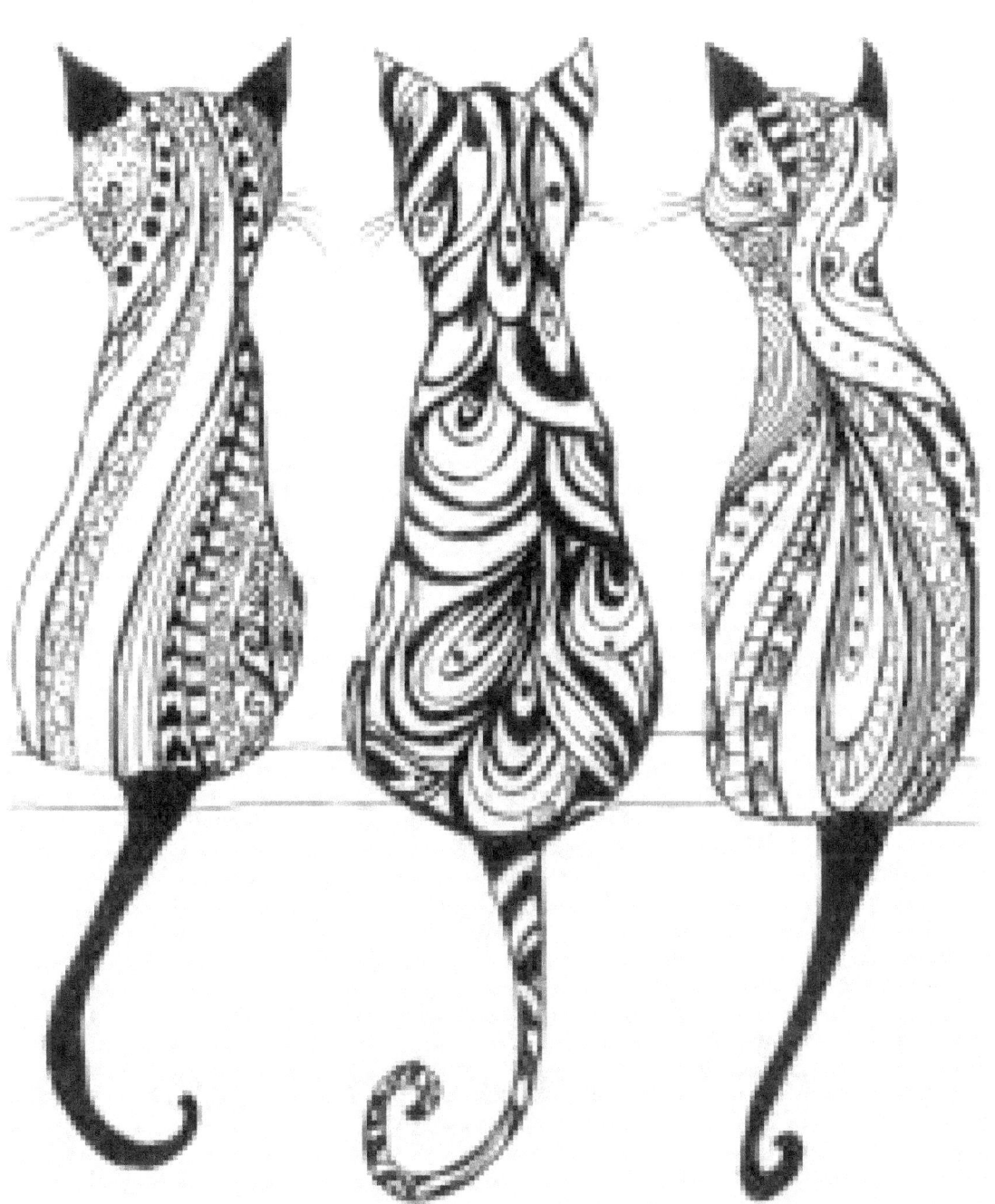

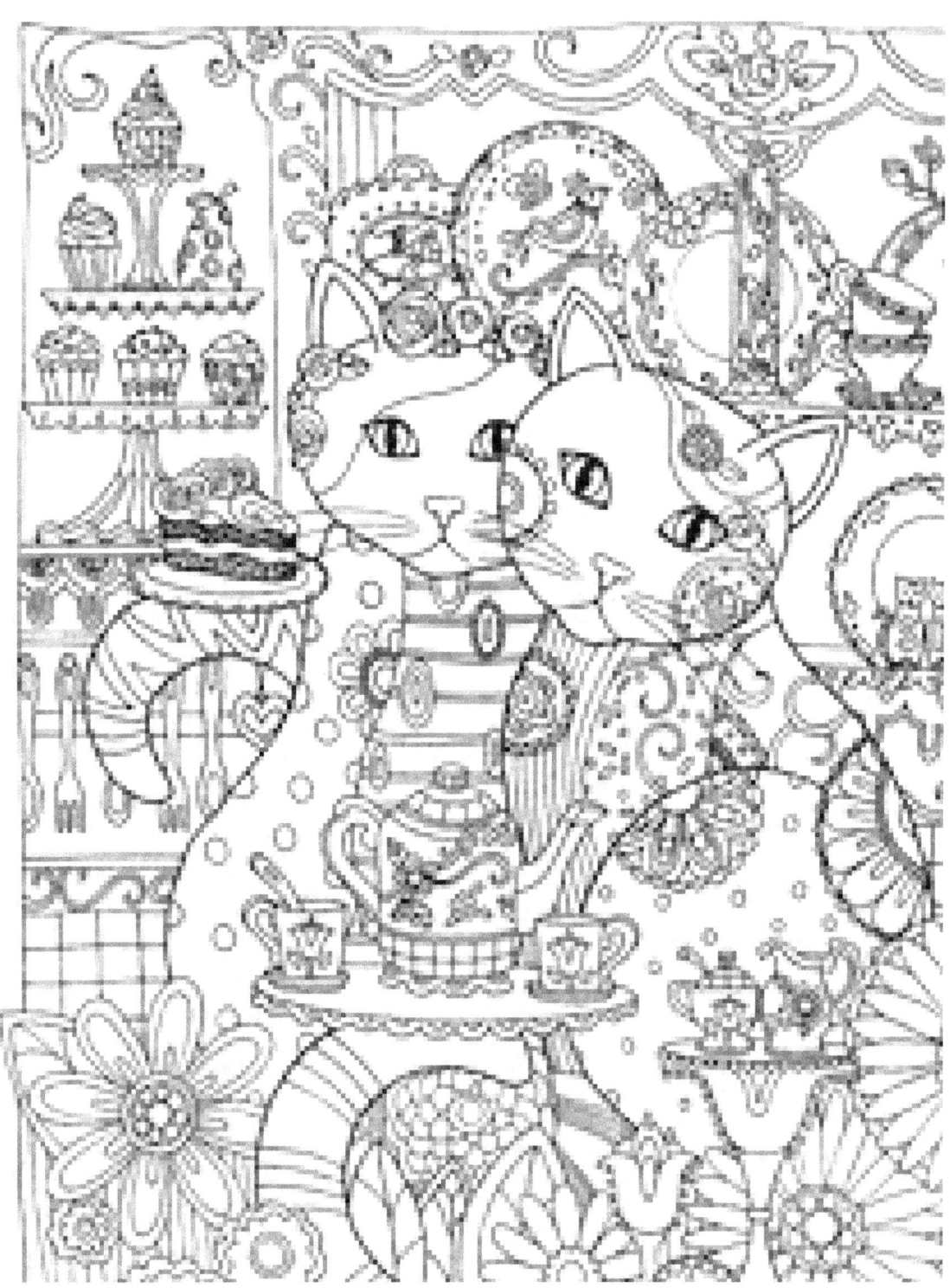

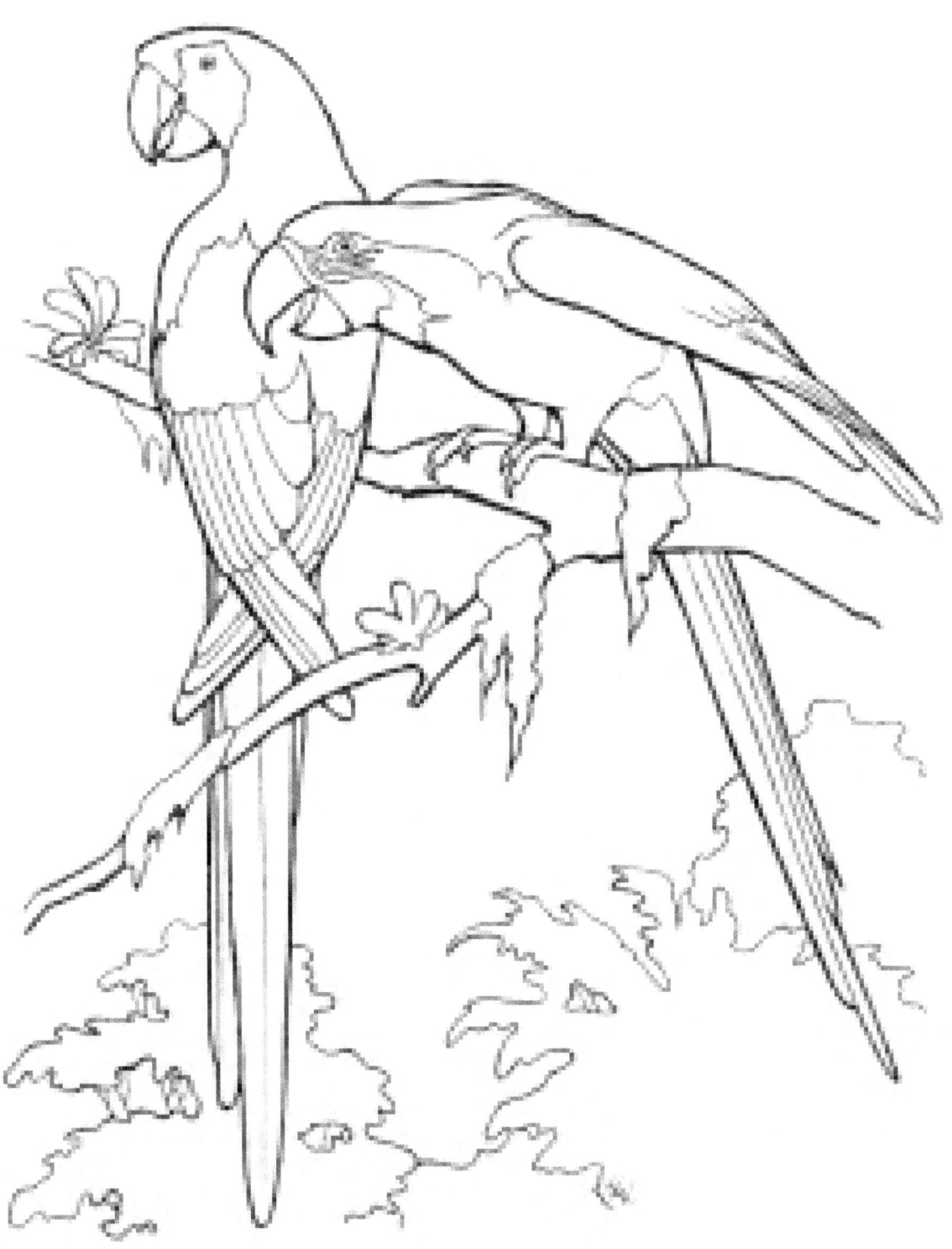

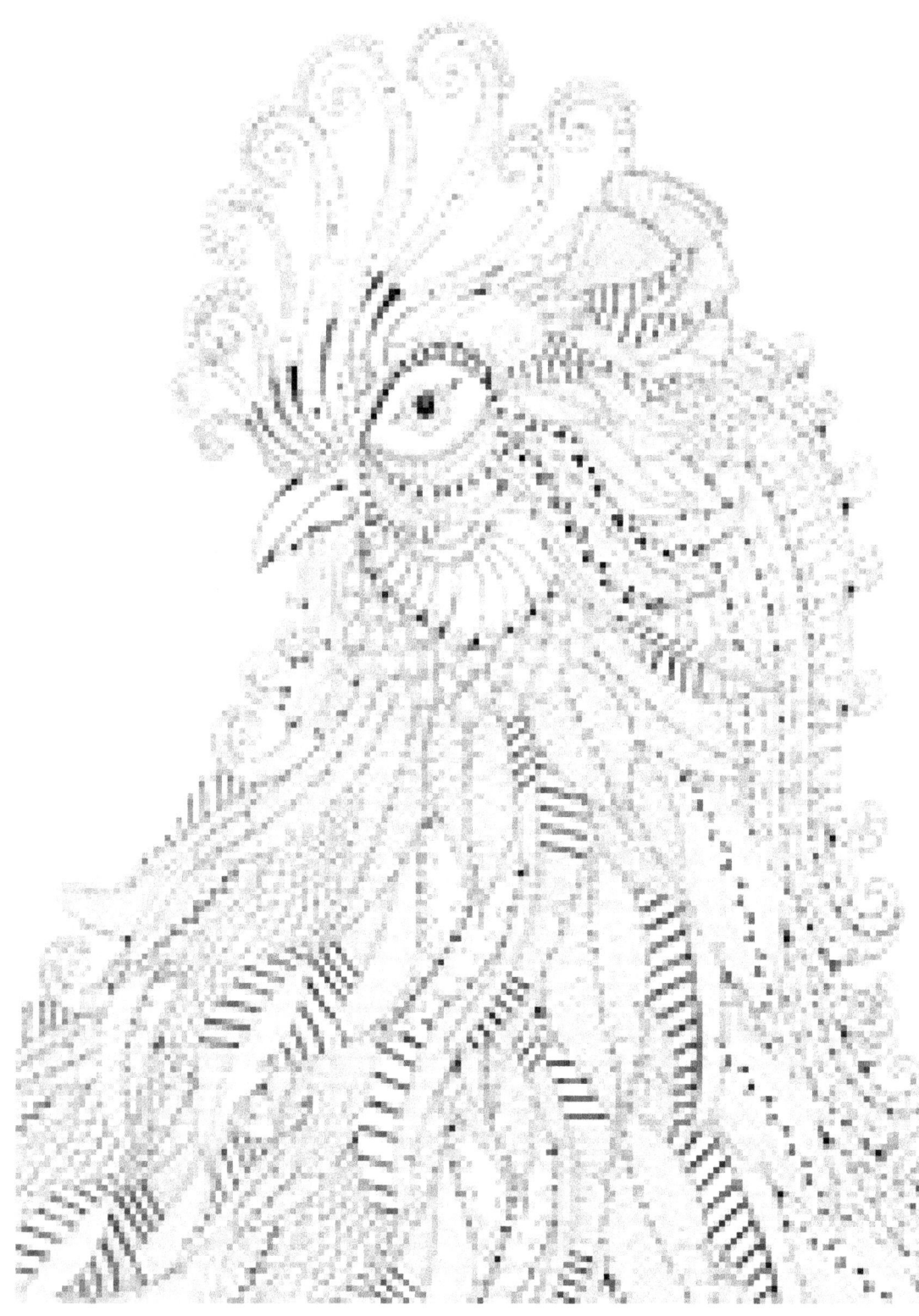

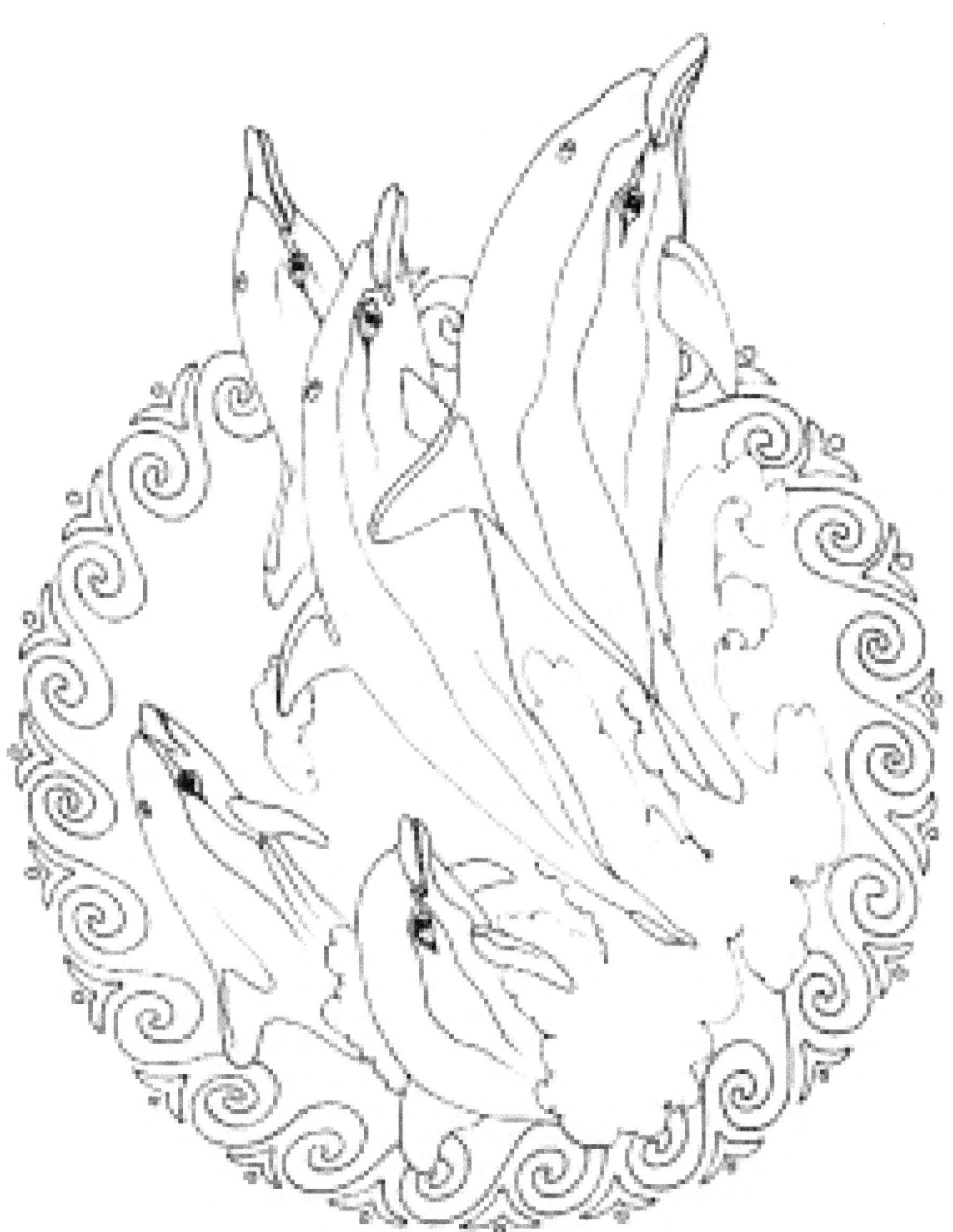

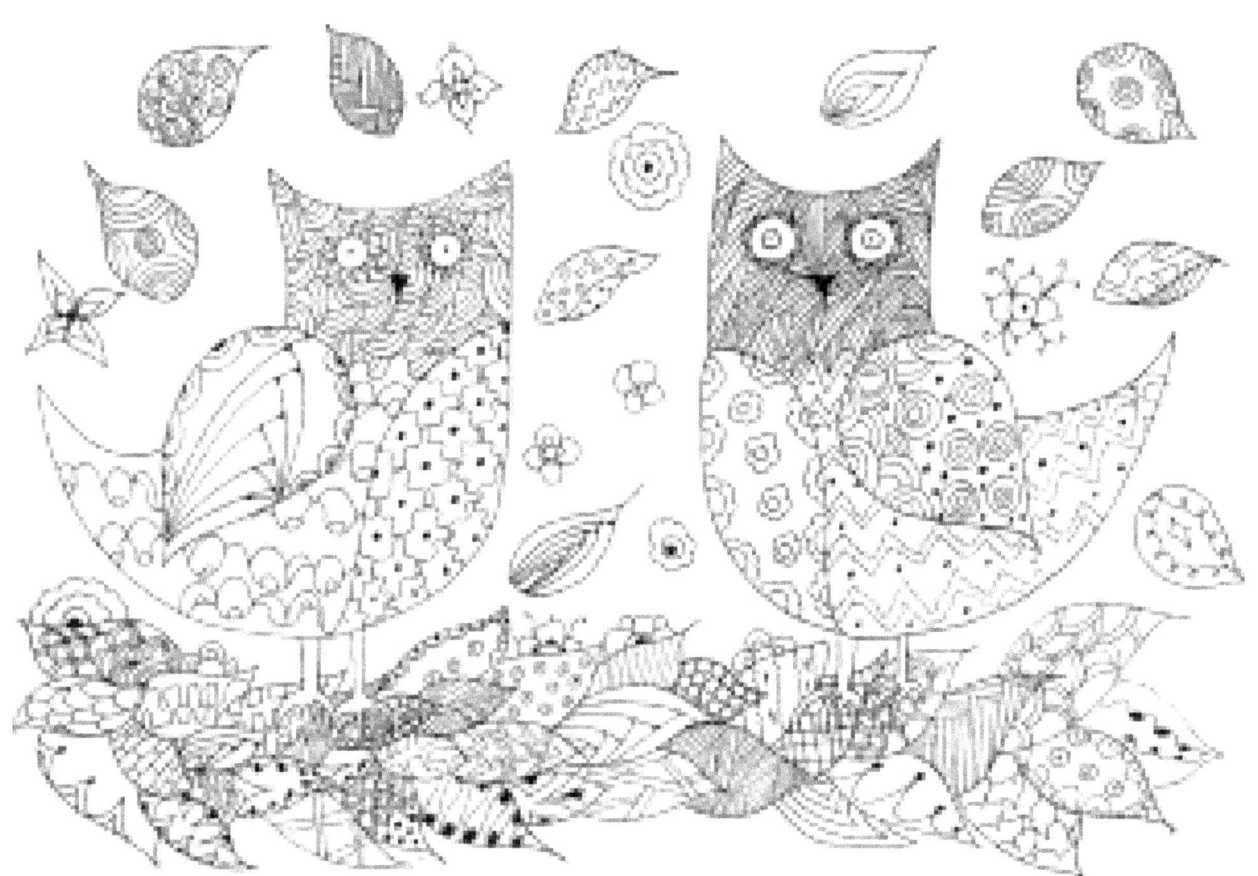

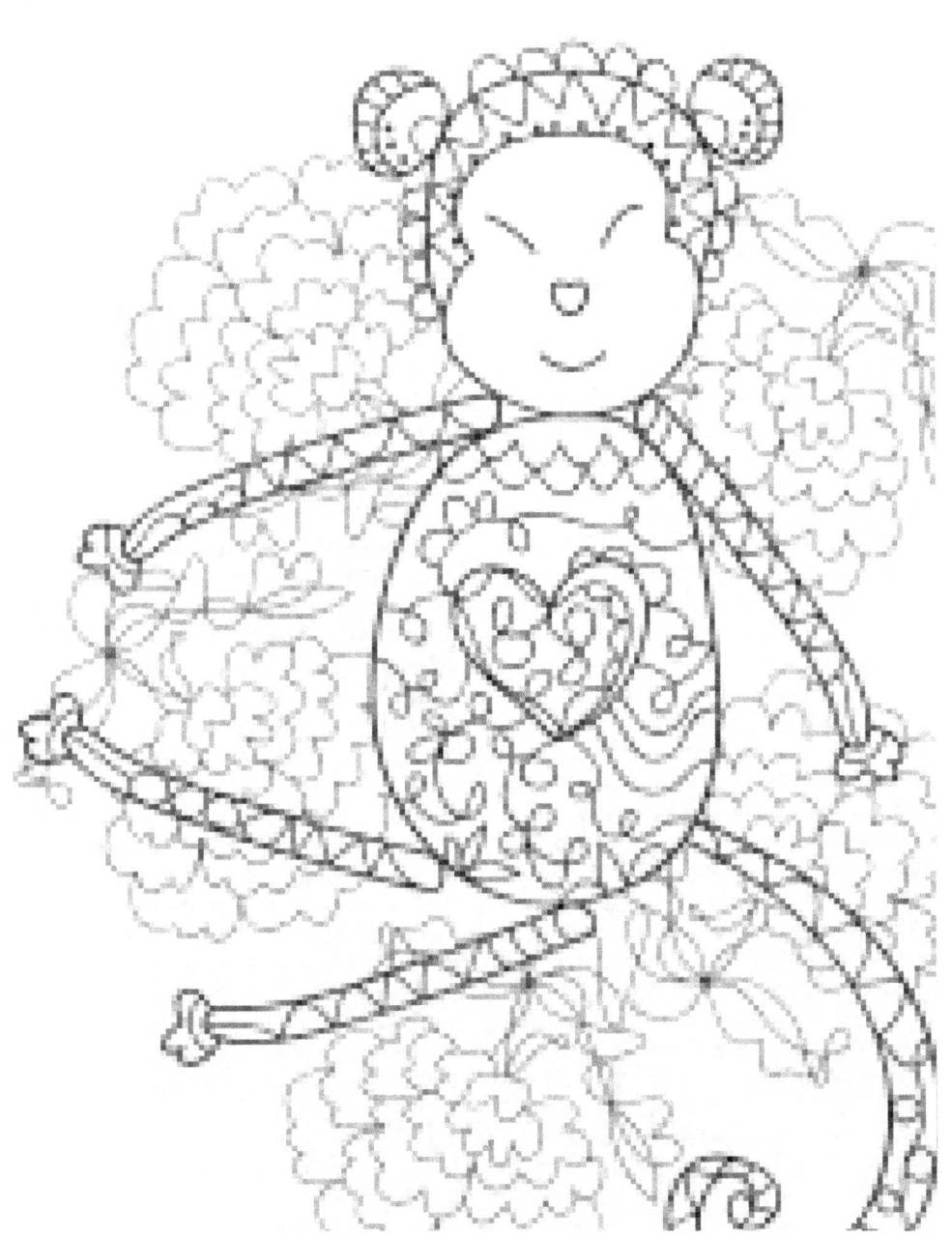

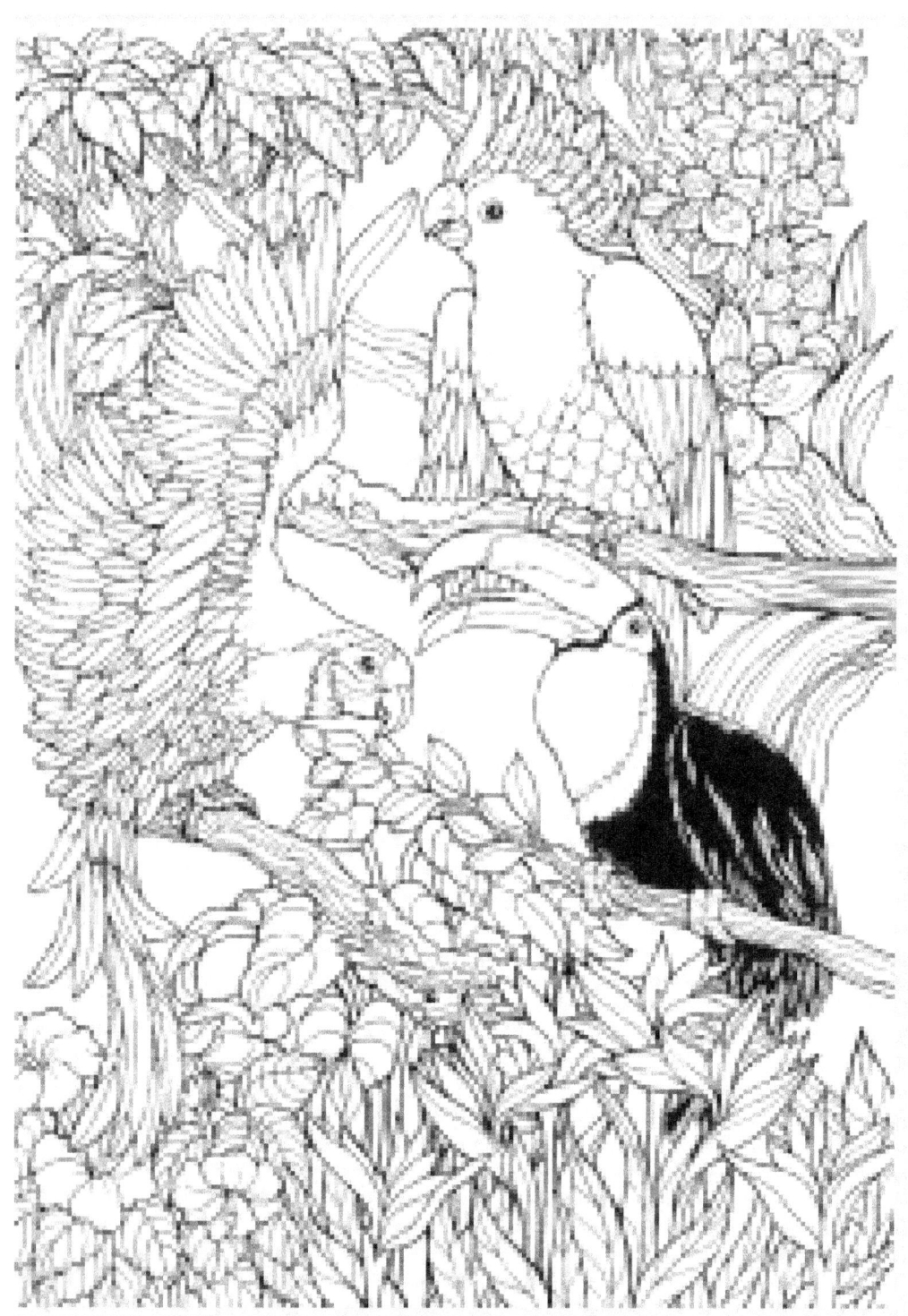

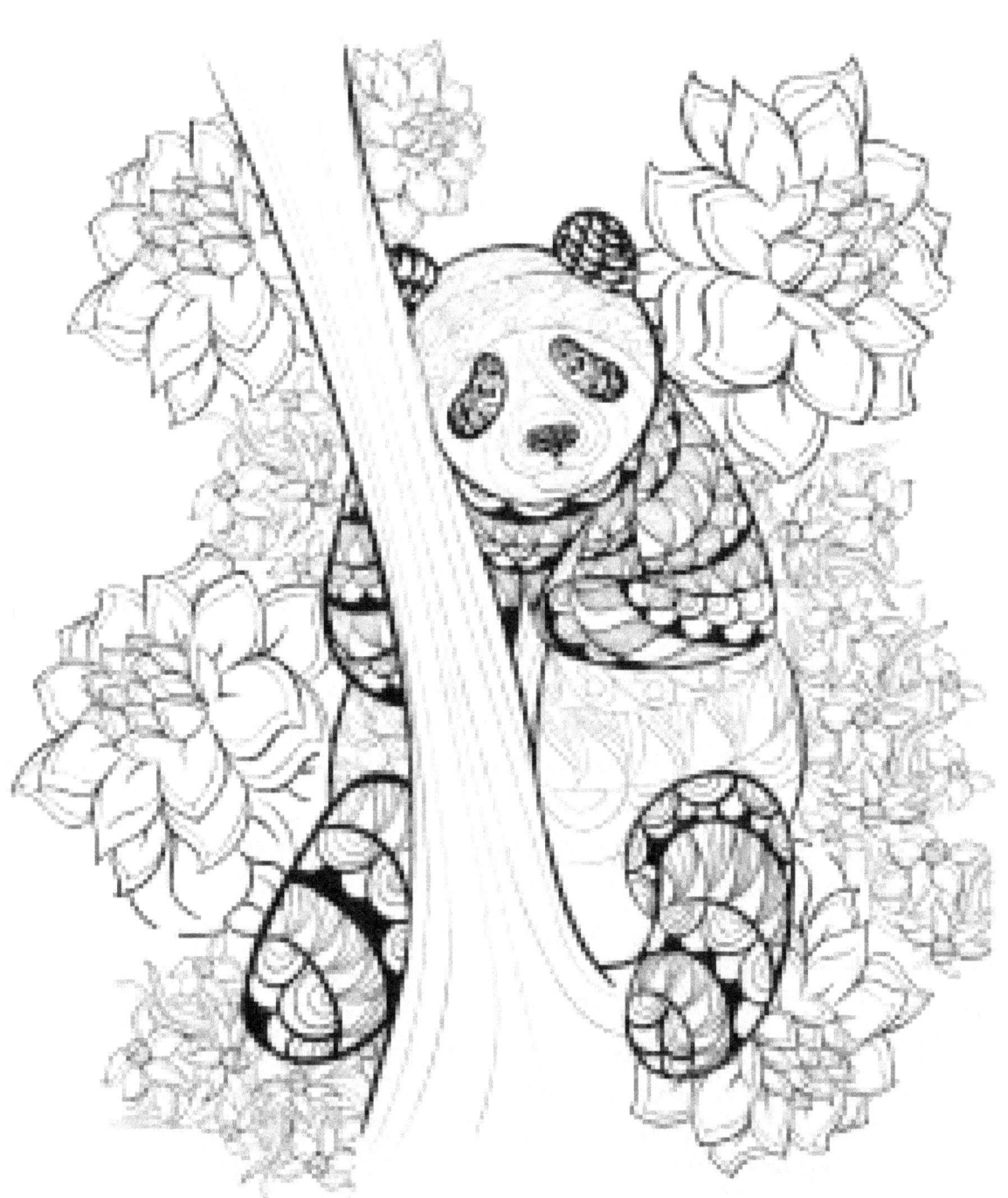

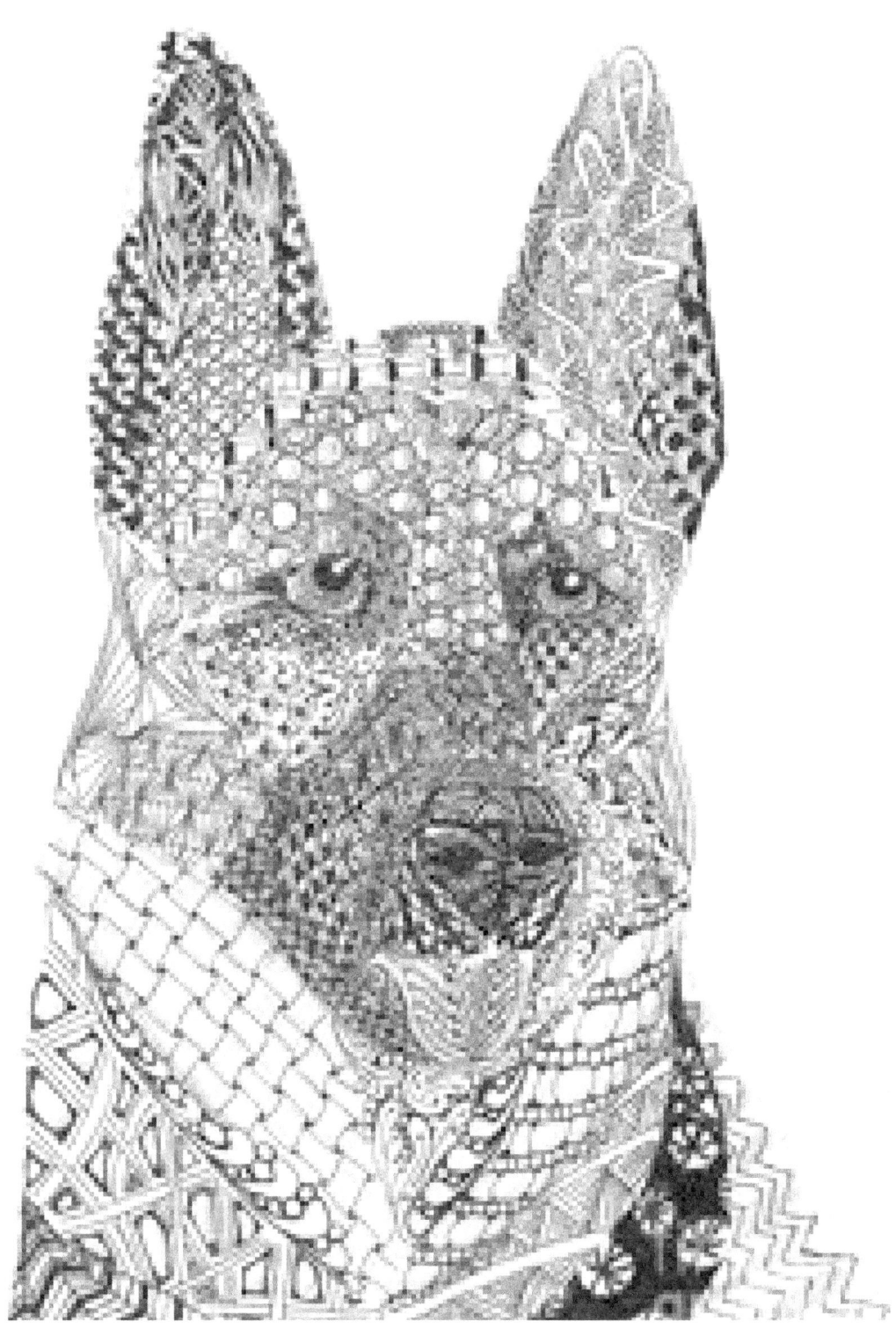

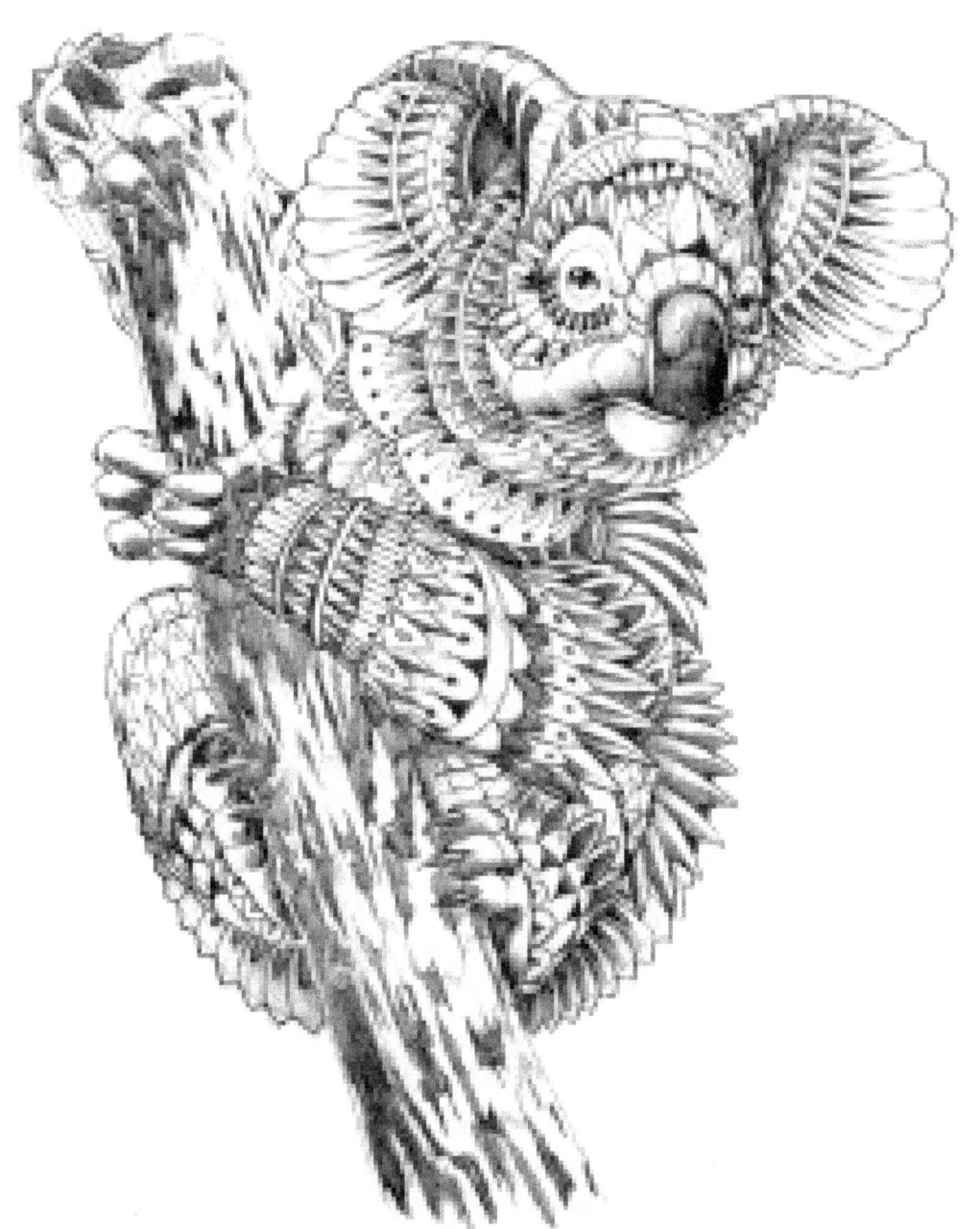

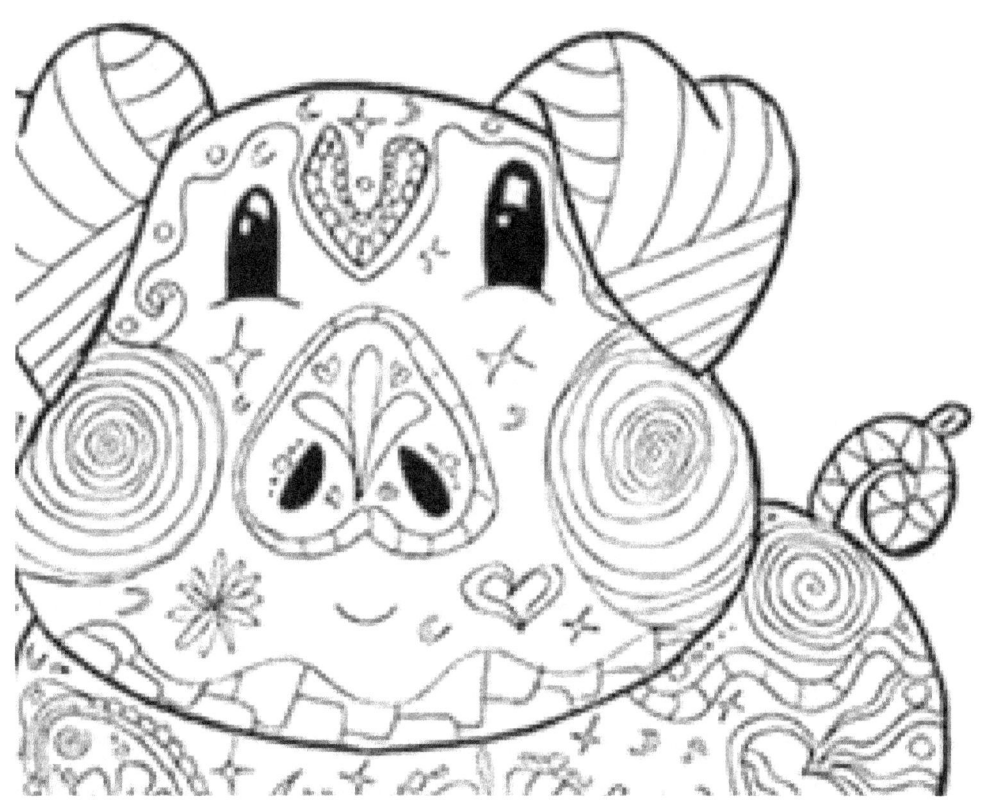

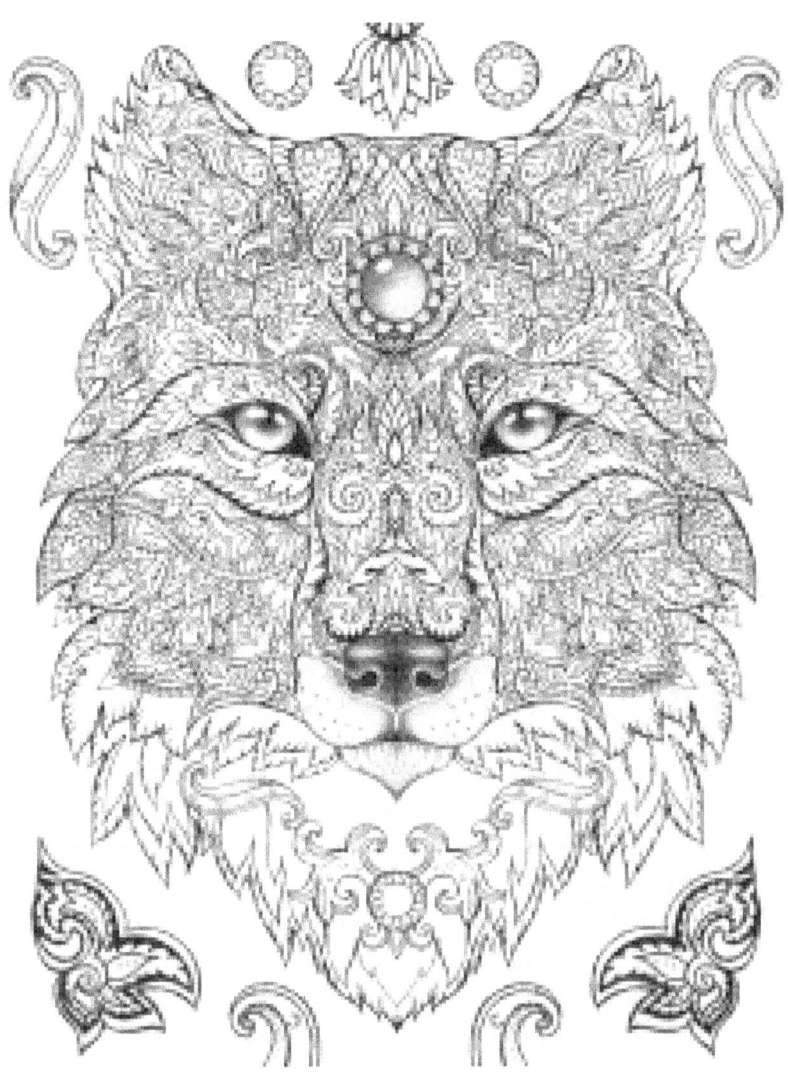

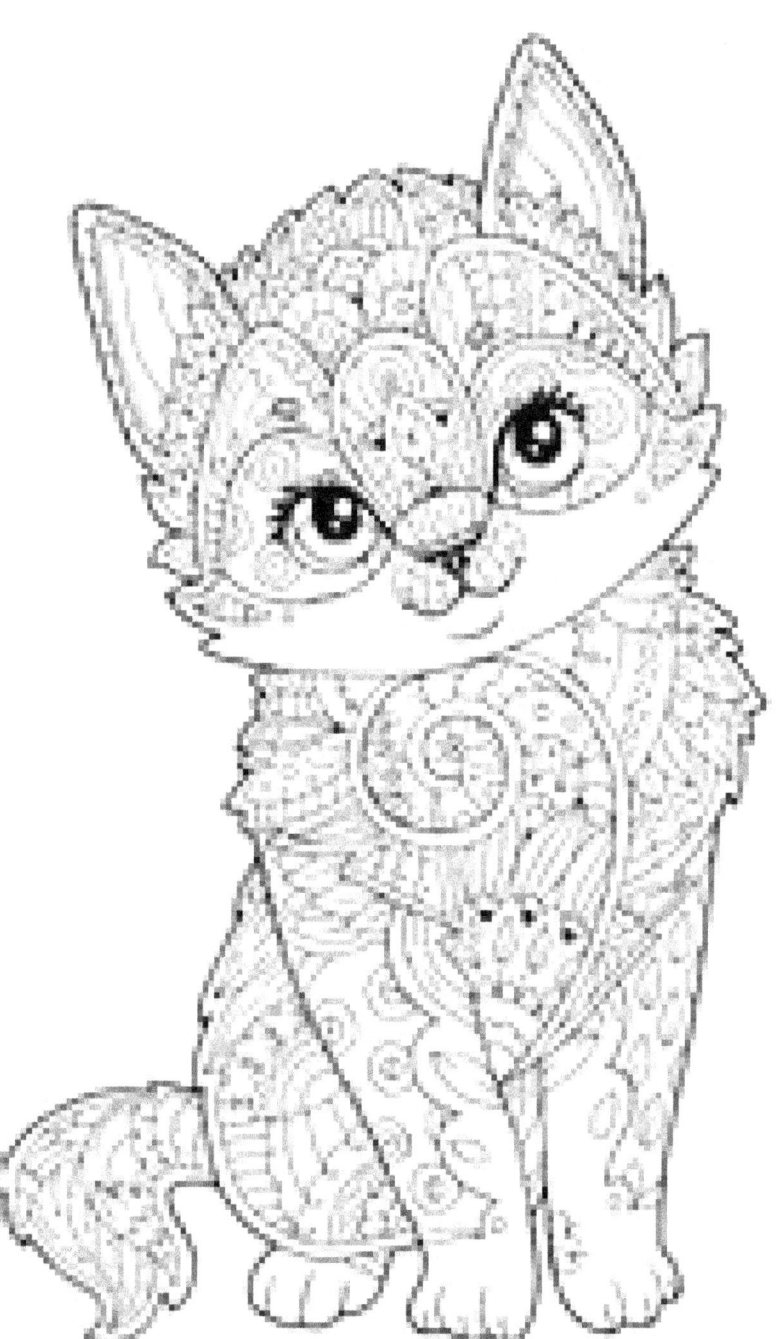

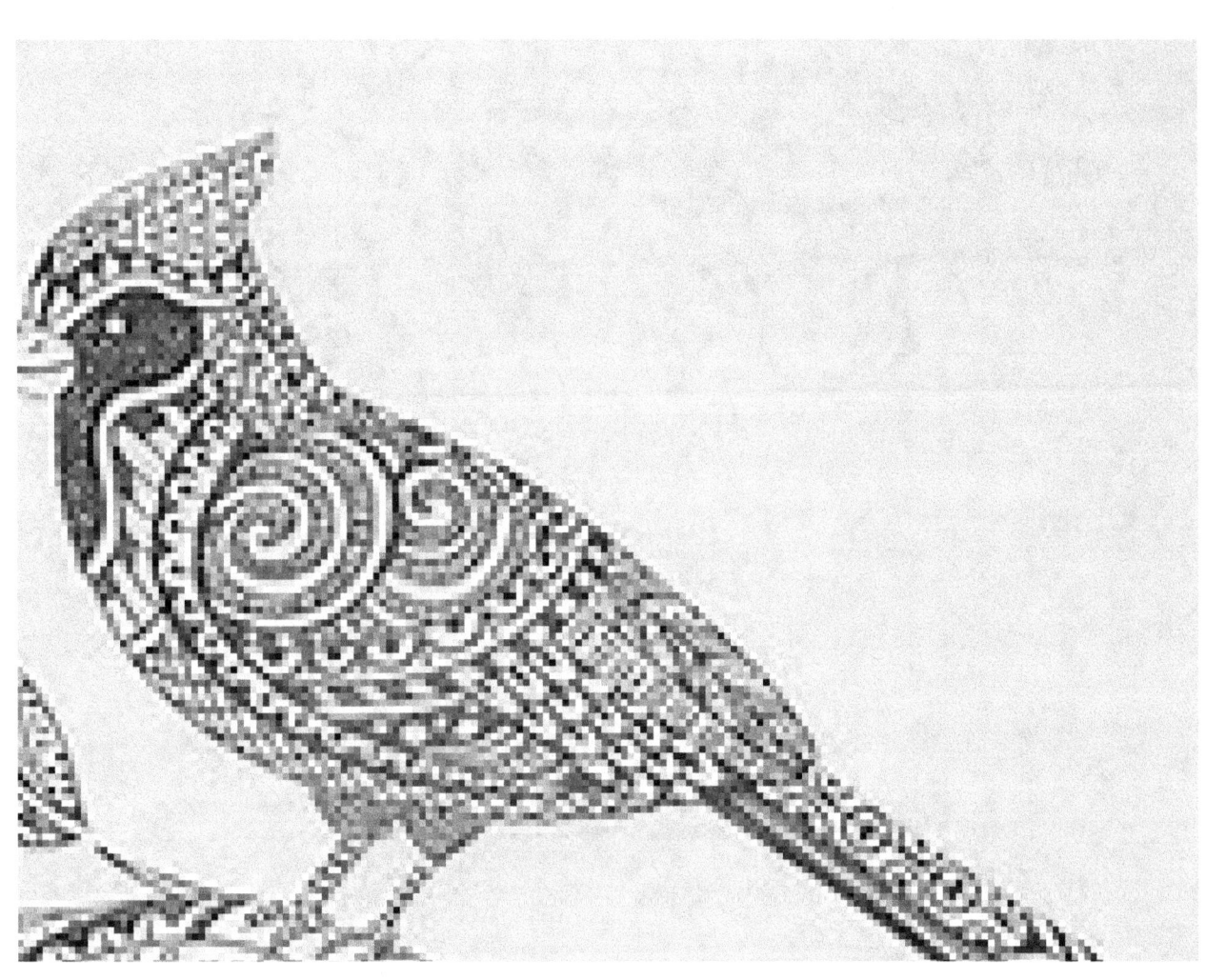

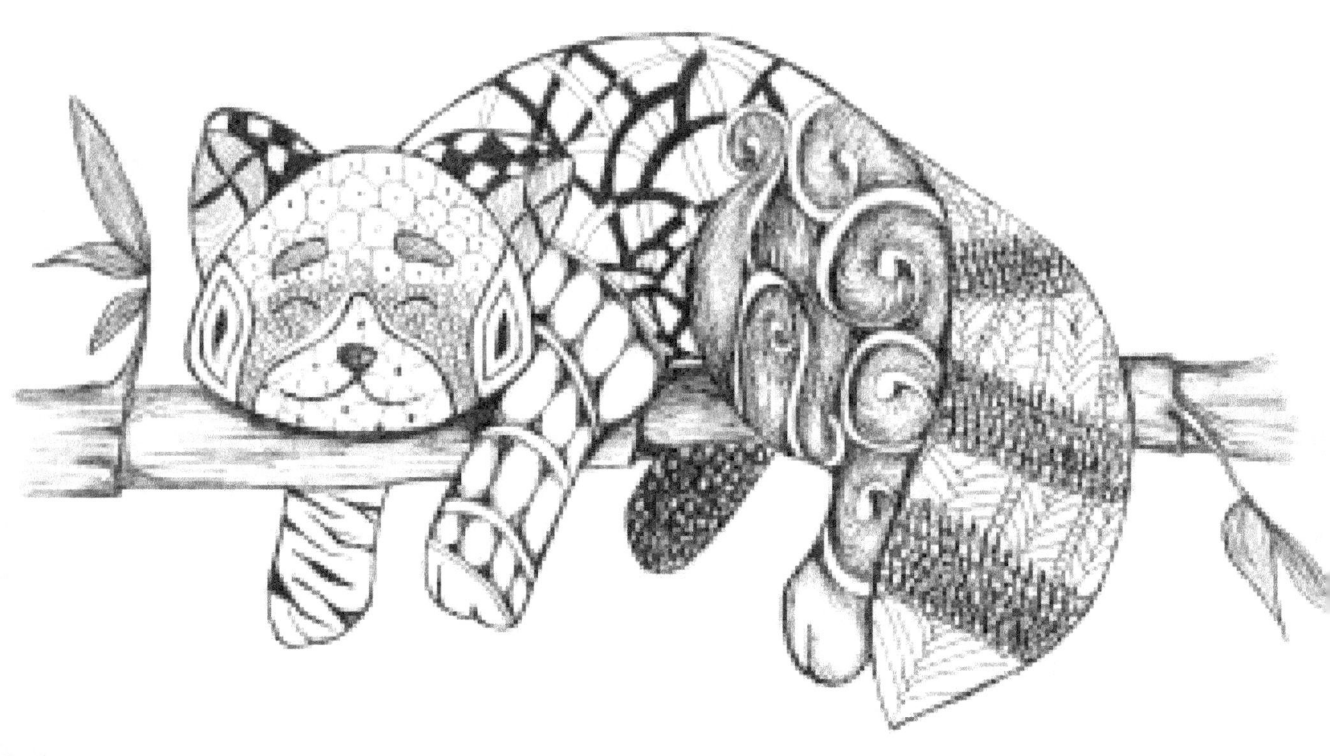

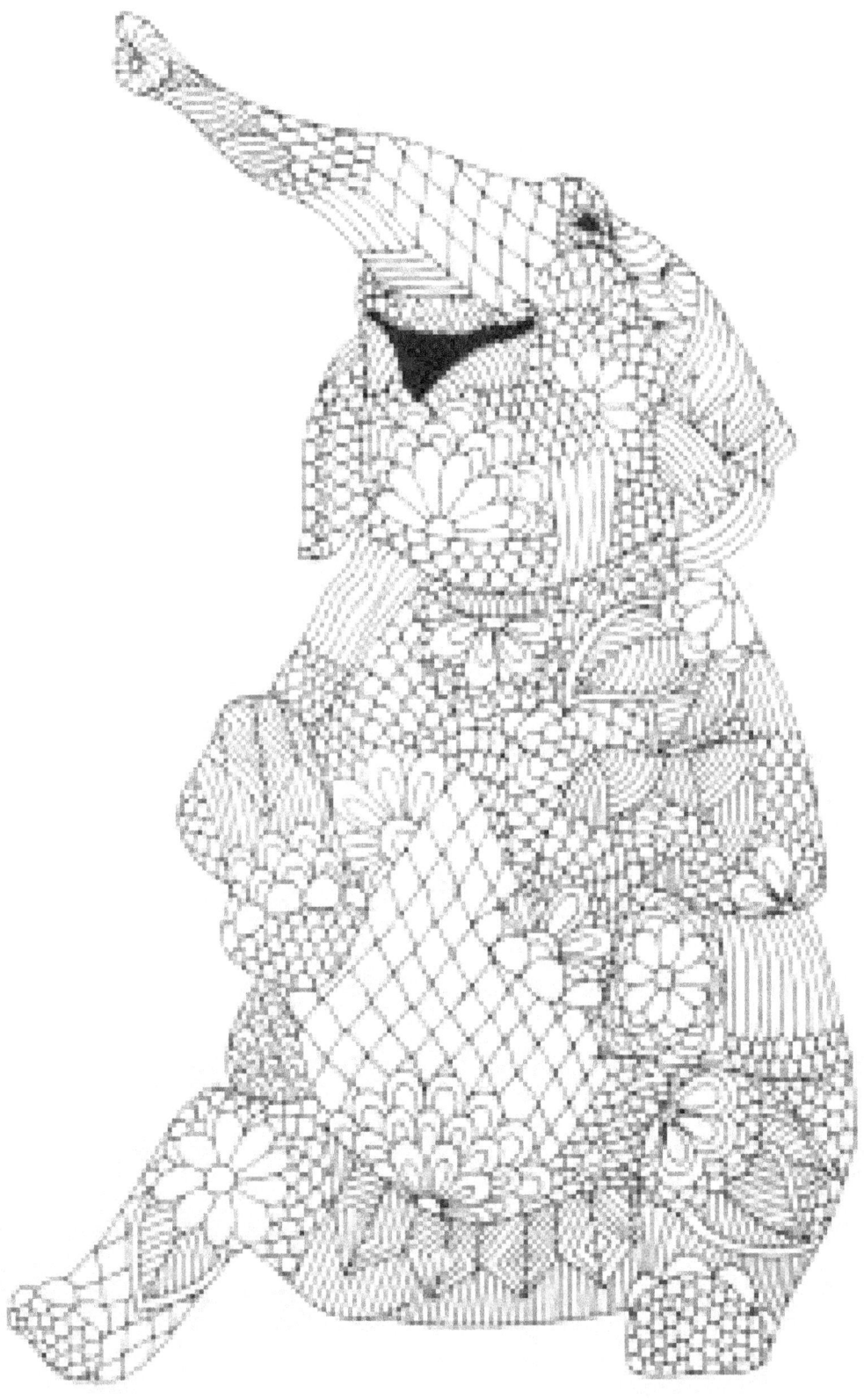

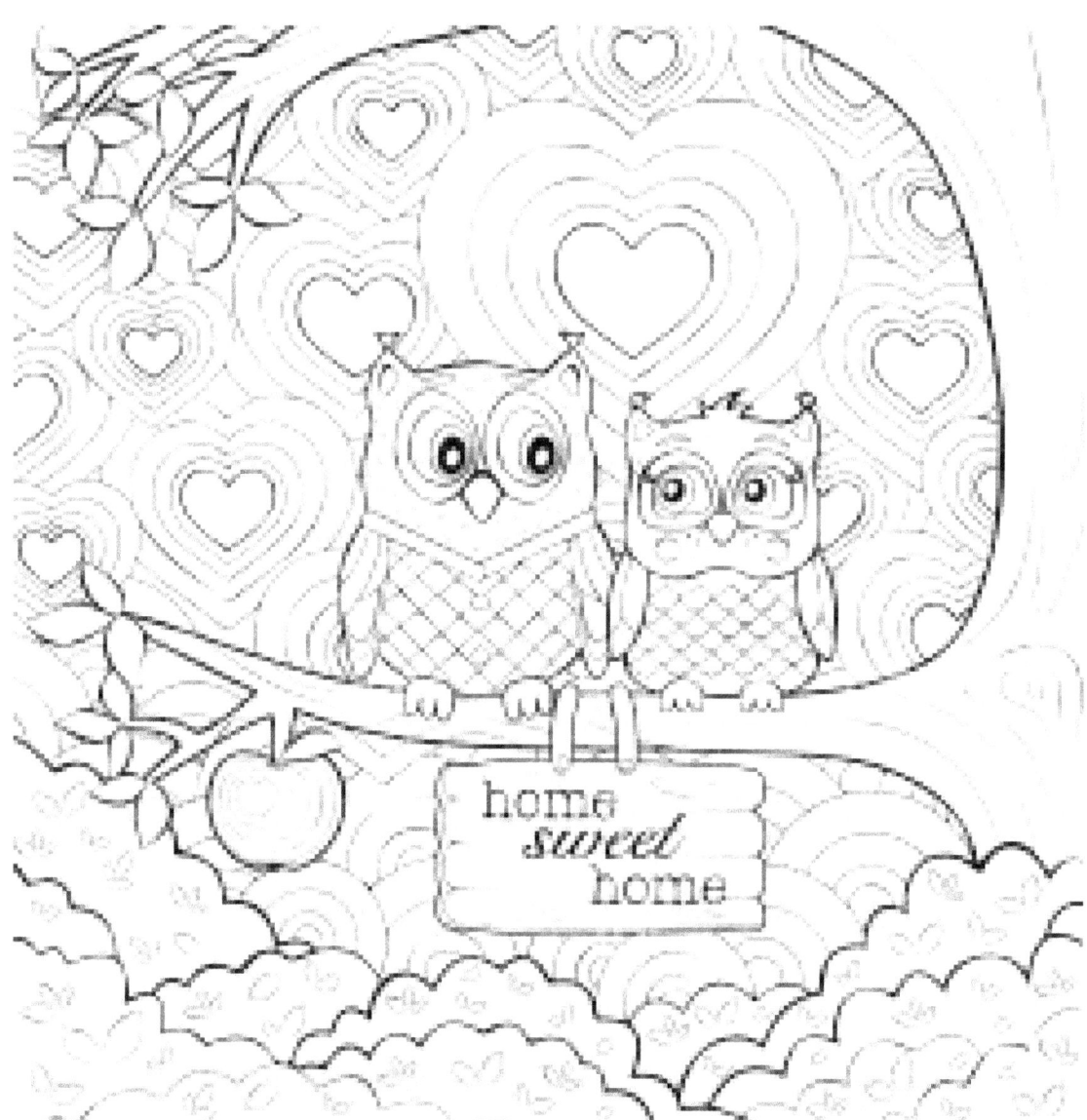

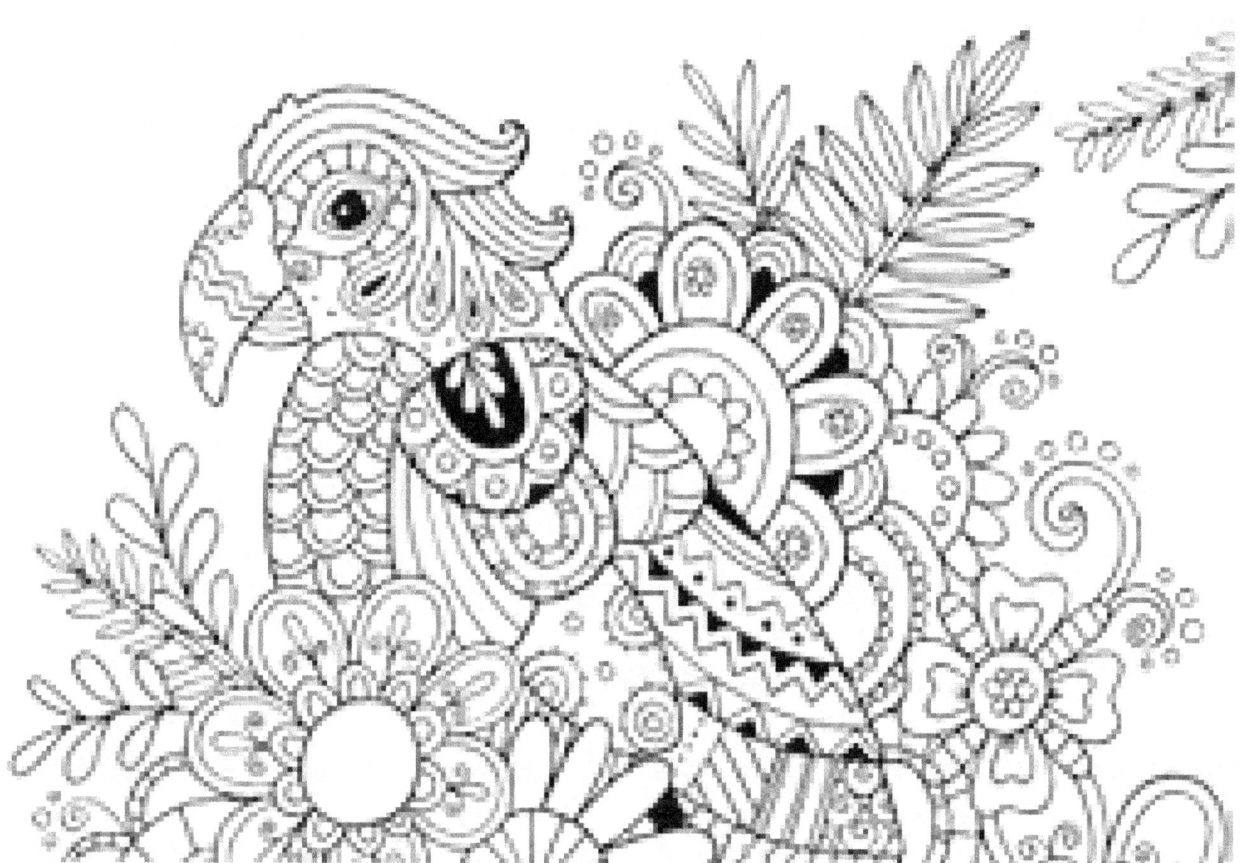

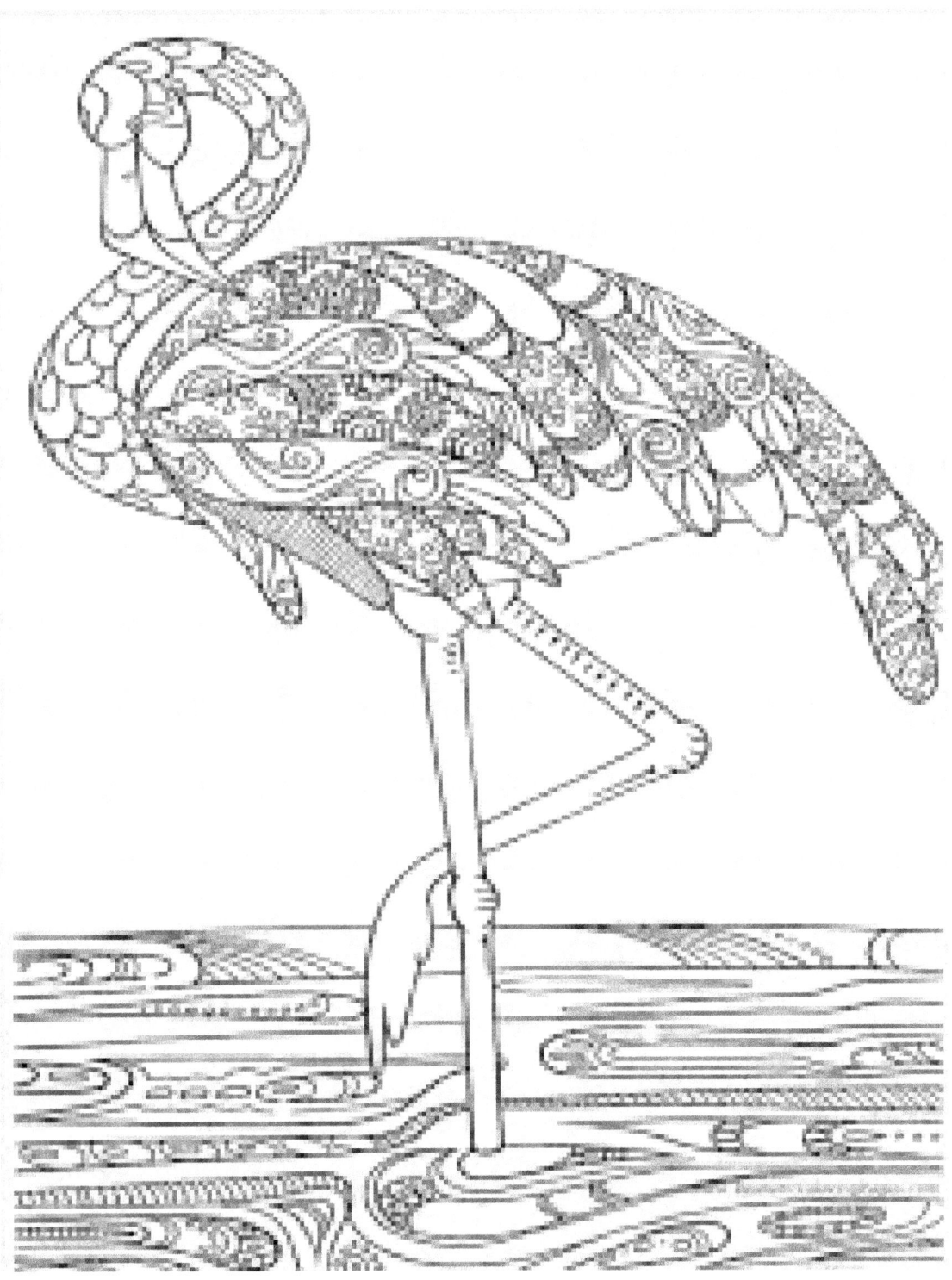

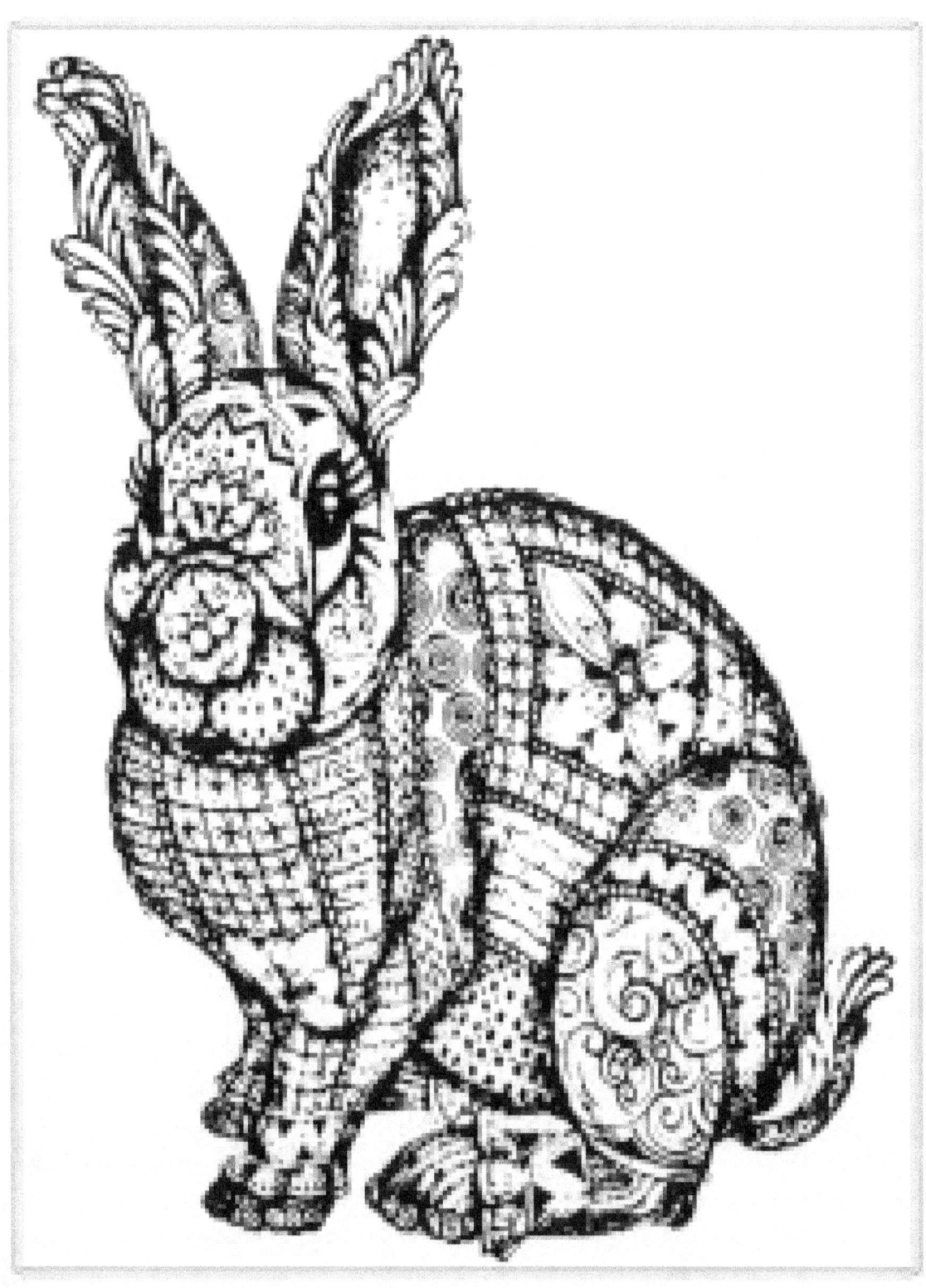

www.ingramcontent.com/pod-product-compliance
Lightning Source LLC
Chambersburg PA
CBHW081123240526
45470CB00019B/2928